How We Can Stop
Promoting

Autism

in Our Children

2nd Edition

Alison Brooks, ND

The publisher and the author make no representations or warranties with respect to the accuracy or completeness of the contents of this work and specifically disclaim all warranties, including without limitation, warranties of fitness for a particular purpose. No warranty may be created or extended by sales or promotional materials. The advice and strategies contained herein may not be suitable for every situation. This work is sold with the understanding that the publisher and author are not engaged in rendering medical or other professional services. If professional assistance is required, the services of a competent professional should be sought. Neither the publisher nor the author shall be liable for damages arising herefrom. The fact that a product, organization, or website is referred to in this work as a citation and/or a potential source of further material and information does not mean that the author or the publisher endorses the products or information the organization or website may provide or recommendations it may make. Further, readers should be aware that internet websites listed in this work may have changed or have disappeared between the time when this work was written and when it is read. Every attempt has been made to indicate a trade or service mark for products that bear them; any omission is unintentional.

How We Can Stop Promoting Autism in Our Children
2nd Edition

Copyright © 2014 by Alison Brooks, ND

1st Edition, Copyright © 2011 by Alison Brooks, ND

Hundredth Shire Publishing, LLC
HundredthShire.com

ISBN-13: 978-0-9895435-3-8
ISBN-10: 0989543536

Testimonials and Letters from Parents

I have only the highest regard for this work written by Dr. Alison Brooks. Her scope and breadth of knowledge of nutrition and how it clearly affects the expression and outcome of the spreading epidemic of autism is clearly evidenced in this book. It is a welcome addition to our compendium of knowledge about food and how it affects the health and wellbeing of our children, and all of us.

Dr. Michael Aronson, MD

In this short work, Dr. Brooks encapsulates the core actions required to bring a child out of the depths of autism, regardless of where he or she may fall on the spectrum. Her principles are sound and methods are scientific. "If you're not testing, you're guessing," is a mantra of hers that I have adopted. Testing then knowing, planning then acting. It seems so simple, yet has profound results. Dr. Brooks' stepwise progression is built on solid ground.

Robin D. Ader, Executive Director
Innovative Health Foundation, Inc.
IHF is a 501(c)(3) organization funding treatments for autism and other psychological, neurological, and learning disorders for children of families in financial need.

Letters of Praise from Parents
for Dr. Brooks' Protocols described herein.

Dear Dr. Alison,

When we started out "A" was prone to Gran Mal seizures. She had an aggressive nature: hitting people, throwing objects, etc. She was unable to interact with other children. She spoke her own language and did not give eye contact when spoken to.

To remind you, before we started supplements and A's diet, for a long time she had been functioning at the developmental stage of a child 16 to 18 months old. Her vocabulary included about 10 words, some echolalia and extensive jargon. And she could understand 20% to 25% of speech spoken by others. Her self-injurious and assaultive behavior, as well as behavior showing extreme resistance when demands are placed upon her, were terrible and she had difficulty with social interactions.

There was significant improvement since we started on your program with supplements and diet changes. First, there was quick improvement after the first two months on the program. As you remember, A has moved from the 18 to 22 months development functioning stage with significant improvement in all the areas including expressive and receptive speech, behavior and social interactions.

Now, A is entering a developmental stage of a child 22 to 24 months. Her vocabulary includes about 50 words, as well as the two-word phrases. Now, she can understand about 50% of the speech spoken by other people. A's self-injurious and assaultive behavior has been improved about 50%. As noted by her therapists, her behavior showing extreme resistance when demands are placed upon her has been improved about 50%. Her difficulty with social interactions has also been improved. For example, every day we see less and less of A appearing aloof and indifferent to other people or making odd, and/or naive social approaches.

Thanks,
EK, Atlanta, GA

Dear Dr. Alison,

I just want to express my deep gratitude for the care you bestowed upon my daughter, G. As you know, we were facing major concerns for her frequent bouts of Asthma, coupled with suicidal thoughts. Your ability to listen with compassion and masterfully get to the 'root cause' of all these issues, was remarkable. G, with consent from our MD, was able to wean off of long term inhalers, and her moods/disposition improved rapidly with your supplements and nutritional guidance.

I am very thankful that my friend referred us to you!

Blessings,
SP, Atlanta

* * *

Dear Dr. Alison,

My husband and I are THRILLED with the positive results we see in our son, C. After hearing over and over again that there is nothing further that can be done for our child, we were in a mental place where hope was fast dwindling. Thankfully we were told about PSI and you!

Although the labs and the supplements were expensive, and the dietary changes were a struggle, you helped guide us and motivate us to hang tight and look forward to the light at the end of the tunnel. Indeed, we are happy we persisted. Within 1 month, we started to see positive changes in C's behavior and overall demeanor. Now, 6 months later we know without doubt, that C will grow to be a happy, productive person. And we could not have done it without your expertise. We will continue with the program as it has helped our entire family.

Sincerely,
AP, Atlanta, GA

Dear Dr. Alison,

I just wanted to share my gratitude for your services and the staff of PSI. As you know, we came to you with much skepticism and as a last effort for our son, J.T. He had been undergoing various therapies (Speech, OT, Neuro-feedback) and although there were some improvements, J.T. began to slip backwards with ability to focus and interact with others. He also suffered with severe mood swings and lack of appetite. Your straight forward, no-nonsense approach coupled with your innate wisdom, compassion and desire to serve, has gotten J.T, finally, on the road to a positive future!

Although this path is not easy, and we endured some rocky roads in getting J.T. to eat and take the supplements according to the program, your patience and cheer-leading helped immensely in the success we are seeing and are overjoyed in announcing.

We are getting the word out in referrals.

God Bless You,
Alpharetta, GA

Dr. Alison,

Thank you so much for your continued support and guidance. "A" was diagnosed with Autism at age 3. After two years of various medications that caused severe issues and hearing from the medical doctors that there was no hope, we thankfully heard about you. We are so pleased with the improvements we and our family see and we are encouraged with hope that A can potentially lead a happy, productive life.

We are honest when people ask about what we are doing in that the tests are expensive and the lifestyle changes were difficult at first, but we are so glad that we stuck it out! You, too, were quite honest in all aspects of this journey, and together with what the test results revealed combined with your encouraging hand-holding with keeping us from straying off the diet month to month, A is progressively coming out of his "prison"!

The word needs to get out that there is HOPE and we will help in doing that. We look forward to what is next and we wish you much success. You deserve it!

With Gratitude,
M, J, L and A, Atlanta, GA

To whom it may concern:

When we first contacted Dr. Alison, our then six year old had been ill for several months with multiple viruses including the Swine Flu, Pneumonia, and Bronchitis. In addition, over the years, he had trouble gaining weight and had problems with lack of energy.

Dr. Alison was so wonderful with our son. She knew the right labs to order so that she could create an individualized protocol to heal is body. The labs indicated he had a metabolic disorder. She taught us how to eat certain foods in the right combinations to gain a healthier immune system. In addition, she prescribed natural supplements that in combination with the special diet were able to address his metabolic issues.

Our now healthy eight-year-old is full of energy, and is gaining weight at a steady rate. We are grateful for Dr. Alison's expertise and her genuine compassion and concern for our son's well-being. She has changed our lives.

S and T, Atlanta, GA

Dedication

I dedicate this book to all children diagnosed with autism. I believe, through them, humanity has been given a gift: The opportunity to learn how our miraculous body can indeed heal itself if given the right medicine. This powerful medicine is called wholesome food. Through these children, families have been able to heal in ways beyond expectations by going back to basics, making lifestyle adjustments, and simplifying life in general. These children are our greatest teachers.

I also dedicate this book to my daughter, Zoe, by biggest inspiration of all. Through her precocious, innate wisdom, I have learned the art of "tuck and roll" with the life journey. And only through parenthood, would I have been given the unique opportunity to evolve into the kind and compassionate person I choose to be. My love for you, Zoe, is eternal.

Acknowledgements

I thank the following people for their contributions:

Phyllis Marks for encouraging me to write this book, for her endless patience and the time it demanded to turn my ramblings into English.

Dr. David Cantor for offering me the wonderful opportunity to work with autistic children from his practice, Psychological Science Institute.

Scott Sutton for his much needed reassurance that 'Everything is going to work out,' and for his continuing dedication to helping humanity.

Drs. MaryAnn Luckett and Carol Billingsley for their honesty in helping me share my knowledge and not my attitude.

Dennis McInerney for allowing me to pick his wonderful brain throughout the many years I've used Biotics Research Corporation products.

Colleen Pettinati for her willingness and passion in sharing her personal story and the success she has achieved with her two children who were once diagnosed with autism. She offers the much needed hope to many families that are about to embark on their own journey to wellness.

Table of Contents

Foreword to the Second Edition

I write this foreword in support of the main thrust of this book with the medical promise in mind, "Do no harm." *How We Can Stop Promoting Autism* highlights much of what has gone wrong with the foundation of the axiom of growth and development: "We are what we eat." This phrase has come to us via a published works over two-hundred-fifty-years old which informs us that for over two centuries members in the health community have been aware of this important fact.

In my nearly thirty years as a clinician working principally with developmental disorders in children, and as a pioneer researcher exploring the nature of brain function as it relates to aberrations of human performance and development, I am pleased to see that gradually over the years, health professional colleagues have developed an awareness and appreciation for the importance of body biochemistry, not just for general health, but even the more subtle mental health of our future citizens. I was fortunate to have the opportunity to work with early brain-behavior researchers to explore the role of nutrition and environmental pollutants on brain-behavior developmental processes in children over three decades ago. This has caught the interest of the American Psychological Association as evidenced by lead articles in 2013 issues of the *APA Monitor*. Some of this work rides on the coattails of early health prophets such as Rachel Carson who, in her 1962 book, *Silent Spring,* tried to warn us of the lethal juggernaut of increased pesticide use and other neurotoxins invading our world and the potential disruption to our very sense of well-being. Carson's work inspired grassroots movements to help create the Environmental Protection Agency and other efforts aimed at monitoring how aspects of 20th century industry may lead to 21st century negative health consequences. Much of this was also followed up by U-Thant, third Secretary General of the United Nations, during his term from 1966-1971, who among other noteworthy accomplishments, initiated the *United*

Nations Environmental Programme (UNEP) as a result of the concern of the international community to identify the serious consequences of, among other factors, the role of pesticides threatening the future of the world-wide population.

How We Can Stop Promoting Autism brings to light the myth that emerged from the 1950s and 1960s, that with the rapid rise of technology and biomedical sciences, a quick remedy will be available to cure the ills of our lives that hamper the freedoms we enjoy in our pursuit of happiness and well-being.   Dr. Brooks highlights for the reader how the trappings of some of the quick fixes, without careful thought and study, has led us to a world of not only malnutrition but a form of neurotoxicity that likely has contributed to an epidemic of developmental disorders with autism arguably being both representative and currently with the highest profile. By the CDC's statistics, between 1997 and 2008, developmental disorders incidents have increased to approximately 17% in the United States, with Autism leading the pack of specific syndromes with an increase of almost 290%![1] This is based on data over just one decade. Autism Spectrum Disorders has become the poster child, in a manner of speaking, largely because as a disorder, it highlights the failure of modern medicine to quickly remedy the problems with some quick-fix medications that can offset its deleterious symptoms effectively (something which was not so apparent in ADHD disorders). If this is any indication of the rise to be expected in future decades, the United States is headed for a population of disabled adults, extremely limited in their ability to contribute to society in levels unprecedented by any society in the history of civilization.

Fortunately, there have been positives in the growth and developmental of biomedical technologies in our understanding of how cellular processes need to function in order to optimize the workings of the myriad of networks that make up human physiology

---

[1] Based on posted statistics at http://www.cdc.gov/features/dsdev_disabilities/

and brain function. We are now able to measure and quantify aspect of biochemistry and of neurofunctional status, and have begun to realize how such measures are strongly correlated to human performance and behavior. We are on the precipice of understanding non-medicinal methods to alter and improve aspects of brain functioning to improve human behaviors and performance. However, we should not miss the biggest point being made by Dr. Brooks' treatise, that as long as children need to eat, they will be influenced by what they consume and what they are exposed to with either negative or positive consequences.

Despite advances in technology, we still have some simple controls and have a choice. Hopefully, with texts like this, we can make informed decisions and begin to turn the tide that is washing away the brightest future for our children.

David S. Cantor, Ph.D.
January, 2014

Autism — a Brief History

Recorded by a scribe of Martin Luther in 1566, is the account of a twelve-year-old boy whom the cleric diagnosed as being possessed by the devil. Based on the description, the boy most likely had autism; this is the earliest record of the syndrome. Another incidence surfaces in the record of a 1747 court case in Scotland, and in 1798 a feral child was discovered who, from the detailed notes of a medical student who attempted treatment, showed several signs of autism.

In 1910, the term "autism" was coined by Eugen Bleuler, a Swiss psychiatrist, from *autos*, a Greek working meaning "self." He had conflated the symptoms with those of schizophrenia. He assigned the term based on his observation of "autistic withdrawal of the patient to his fantasies, against which any influence from outside becomes an intolerable disturbance."

The Viennese psychiatrist, Hans Asperger first used *autism* in its modern sense in 1938. Leo Kanner of Johns Hopkins Hospital used it in the 1940s when there were only twelve diagnosed cases of autism in the United States.

Autism and schizophrenia remained linked in many researchers' minds until the 1960s. For the following twenty years, research into treatments for autism focused on medications and behavioral change techniques including pain and punishment. Then, in the 1980s and 1990s, the role of behavioral therapy and the use of highly controlled learning environments became the primary treatments for many forms of autism and related conditions.

From the first modern diagnoses of autism with just a dozen cases in the 1940s, we now face hundreds of thousands of children, some already into adulthood, who are confined in their childlike psyche, limited in their ability to function or communicate, and totally dependent for their survival.

Perhaps there's more we can do.

Introduction

Families affected by autism are thrown into chaos and despair. Parents ask, "How did this happen to my child?" To date, no one has provided a definitive answer as to what causes autism. Although there's much speculation, nothing has been proven scientifically.

The alarming increase of autism in our children over the past decade has led some experts to proclaim that we are in an "autism epidemic." In March 2011, the Centers for Disease Control—the CDC—estimated that one in one-hundred-ten children in America has Autism Spectrum Disorders—ASDs. These are scary statistics, and it's predicted to get worse, growing at an annual rate of ten to seventeen percent.

I have learned from working with autistic children that there are no quick-fix solutions; there is no silver bullet that will make this devastating syndrome go away. Since the first diagnoses in 1943, with only twelve reported cases, it has taken several generations to hit the statistics released by the CDC in 2011.

I have often wondered how we got from those twelve reported cases to the shocking numbers we see today. I've looked at our society and noted the changes that have taken place over these seven decades. Life has accelerated drastically and we've become accustomed to everything happening fast. I've wondered, could our quick-fix lifestyles *itself* be promoting autism?

In helping parents deal with the devastation of this syndrome, my experience has been that it takes time, tremendous sacrifice, and focused effort to turn the major symptoms around. Quick-fix methods have never achieved the same long-term benefits that I have accomplished with a carefully designed and implemented program.

I believe we must enact persistent lifestyle changes, if we hope to make a lasting impact and stem the autism crisis.

Let me state, up front, that none of what I say is based on scientific evidence, just my observations and the successes of those who have followed my advice.

I ask you to decide for yourself whether it makes sense to you or not. It is my goal to provide you with useful information that will help your child and ultimately your entire family.

At times, I speak of my practice and the approach I have adopted in working with my autistic clients and their parents. Those passages are necessarily in the first person. But I am not alone; throughout North America there are many naturopaths, medical doctors, and other healthcare practitioners that have embraced functional lab testing, a diagnostic method that is discussed in detail later on. I consider this the primary tool to determine the nutritional status of your child, and that knowledge is the gateway to relief.

When selecting a healthcare professional to work with your child, not only are you *allowed* to interview the practitioner to decide if he or she is a good fit for you, it is imperative that you do so. Ask if they use functional lab testing. Ask their experience with this modality. Be certain they have employed these techniques to address autism.

Follow my blog at http://AlternativeMedicineAtlanta.net for more news regarding updated information about autism.

Alison Brooks, ND
Roswell, GA
November, 2013

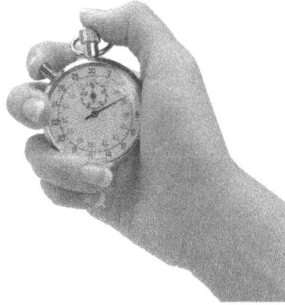

Chapter 1: Our "Quick-Fix Syndrome"

We are privileged to live in a society with so many conveniences. Our lifestyle is coveted around the world. Most of the things we want are at our fingertips. But, there are trade-offs, and the explosion of the fast food industry is one.

While the convenience of fast food has certainly made our lives easier, quick-fix food is well documented as the cause of the alarming increase of obesity in our children. It does not just make us fat, it makes us unhealthy; it contributes no nutrition to grow strong and fend off disease and dysfunction, while it doses young bodies and minds with dangerous chemicals.

Instant Gratification Has Become Ingrained in Our Society

Technology has made it possible to fulfill our desires immediately. It's no wonder that we have developed an attitude that demands instant gratification. I call it the "Quick-Fix Syndrome." This expectation has devastating effects on our health and that of our children.

We want a pill that makes symptoms go away. There's not much emphasis on getting to the root cause of disease where we could eliminate it altogether and avoid the need for medications. With the ever-increasing stress that is rampant in our lives, it is much easier to rely on drugs that bring quick relief so that we can make it through another of our fast-paced days.

My vision is to make Americans, and all those that follow our lifestyle pattern, become more aware of how our daily actions are having a profound impact on our health. I imagine a society where we accept accountability for our own health and take steps to ensure that we never fall ill due to poor choices. I hope for a society where health insurance is a rarely used safety net.

What Does the Quick-Fix Syndrome Have to Do with Autism?

It is not uncommon for parents to be asked, "Is your child on the spectrum?" And, sadly, just about everybody understands what that means.

I view autism as the worst possible outcome of how we live our lives unaware of the fundamental part that nutrition plays in the health of a child's developing mind. Most people make fast food choices every day without regard to nutrition. It is so easy to buy something that looks like food on the way home, rather than cook. The consequence is the explosion of obesity and other diseases in our children.

The time has come for us to look at what we are doing to our kids. The problem has become huge. If we don't change our habits, and we *must*, it will get worse.

No matter how badly we might want it, or wish for it, there are no quick-fix solutions for autism spectrum disorders.

My Quick-Fix Rant

I am on a quick-fix "rant" because it is my hope that I can help to wake up America. I want to do my part to alert parents to what they are doing to their children. It is easy to blame someone or something *out there*, but only through substantial changes in family lifestyle—which will require sacrifice—can parents eliminate autism.

> Much of the work that needs to be done takes place in the home.

It will take time, energy, commitment and considerable effort. There is no getting around the fact that much of the work that needs to be done takes place in the home, not a doctor's or therapist's office. And this is not an easy task for a family already under the stress of care-giving to an autistic child.

While I know it will be difficult, we have no choice but to go back to food basics. We have to take that first step in changing our lifestyles, if we have any chance of turning this around.

What I See Time and Again

What I witness each time I consult with the parents of an autistic child is heart-wrenching. They are at the end of their ropes and their outlook is bleak. Their children have been sick for a long time without being helped by conventional means. Their lives are in shambles and their families are being torn apart from the strain of coping with the problems attendant to the autistic child. I watch them as they gaze with anguish at the child they love and so desperately want to help. The

> Autism impacts families as much as individuals.

unspoken terror that lives with them is, "Who will take care of my child when I no longer can?"

As best she can, mom manages her child's aberrant behavior while we speak in my office. My questions derive from a symptom-based questionnaire I have developed. A picture of their lives comes into focus. More often than not, it's mom who spends every waking moment of her life caring for a totally dependent child that might be 2-½ to 16 years old and, perhaps, not yet toilet trained.

If there are other siblings, she does not have the time or energy to spend with them, and she is often riddled with guilt because of it. Her options are few; responsibility to her child will never end. In most cases, the child cannot interact with other people or make friends. How many marriages have failed due to this tremendous pressure?

Autism begins in the Gut

In every case, autism spectrum disorder demands lifestyle changes if the child is to be helped. And these changes never involve a quick-fix solution. I won't kid you, it's hard, very hard to make these changes because the initial adjustments require taking food from the child that he probably loves.

The hard part for me is that, initially, what I'm asking puts even more burden on the family. It heaps more responsibility on Mom by asking her to prepare and cook whole food meals. I am aware that most moms are already stressed to the max in just dealing with their autistic child, but there is nothing else that will help.

In the case of autism, food is medicine and medicine is food. We have to start with the food because in every autistic case I've encountered, the child has digestive issues: *autism begins in the gut.*

Advanced Meal Planning and Preparation is a Must

It is critical to focus attention on what the child is eating and drinking. There can be no fast food, no boxed or canned food. No dairy or soy, wheat, or refined and chemically produced sugars. You cannot feed your child anything with unknown ingredients. The only way to ensure this is to go back to basic meal planning and preparation using nutritious whole foods.

A whole food is one which is close to nature: fresh organic fruit and vegetables, hormone and antibiotic free meats, and other goodies that will be described later.

Of course, there will be times when you won't be able to stick to the program. Just get back on track as quickly as possible. If you do the very best you can, it will go a long way toward helping your child.

It will be necessary to plan for your child's meals in advance. This is the *only* way to control what goes into his mouth. In consultation, I get specific: "If it can't rot, your child can't eat it. Of course eat it before it rots." Simply, your child must eat whole, live foods. No ice cream or chocolate milk. I provide a list of appropriate foods to get started. I let parents know I am willing, if necessary, to hold their hands every step of the way.

Most often, as I consult, parents are dismayed; it sounds overwhelming. What I'm advising involves a lifestyle changes that will wreak havoc on their lives. They already don't have enough time as it is and I'm asking them to add even more—but it can't be helped. I'm truthful with parents in explaining that there is no way other than to eliminate non-nutritious foods from their child's diet. It's a necessary step to get to the root cause and eliminate the symptoms and help their child. Again, the mantra: *There are no quick-fix solutions.*

Implementing Changes is a Step-by-Step Process

Change takes time. Everything cannot be done immediately. It may take six months before you implement all dietary and lifestyle changes. But if you take one step at a time, you will get there. It's hard to say "No" to your child when they are asking for something that makes them happy. Sometimes it's heartbreaking, but what you have to grasp is that with perseverance positive results can be seen in as few as thirty days. Commitment to program-compliance is the key to success.

It comes down to this:

- Do you want to spend the rest of your life dragging your sick child from one doctor to another with no results?

- Do you want to have to pay for tutoring your special needs child for the rest of the time he goes to school?

- And what about the high price tag for schools specifically designed for autistic kids?

- What will happen to your child when he becomes an adult?

- Would it not be a wonderful thing to finally get the answers that you have been praying for?

- Would it give you hope if you had a definite plan of action that you know will give you the results you seek?

I am not insensitive to the challenges you face: the responsibility of an autistic child and the high price tag that comes with it. The lifestyle changes I'm talking about will invariably cost money. You will have to do functional (biomedical) lab testing to reveal why your child has specific problems, and to identify your child's needs. You will have to select *organic* in many of your food choices. You will have to engage in food planning, and cook your child's meals at home for the most positive results.

> I am not insensitive to the challenges, but you must face them for the sake of your child.

This is the only way a potential healing program can be designed that fits your child's specific needs and has the greatest chance of success.

Let's Wake Up

If we understand what we are doing to future generations through poor food choices, we can implement positive changes. We must be aware of how food affects the health of our children. We must accept that there are no quick-fix solutions for the autism crisis. Then we can take the steps to eradicate it.

Chapter One Summary

1. We are privileged to live in a society where we have so many conveniences.

2. We benefit from having things we want are at our fingertips. But as with everything in life there are positives and negatives.

3. We must become aware of how our fast-paced lifestyles impacts our health. We must be accountable for our health and take steps to ensure that we never forfeit it due to unhealthy food choices.

4. Autism is an outcome of how we have chosen to live. We are unaware of the fundamental part that nutrition plays in the health of our children. Most people make non-nutritional fast food choices every day, rather than cooking at home. The unforeseen consequence is a fast food habit and diseases in our children.

5. We are in an autism crisis and the need for a major wake up call. One in one-hundred-ten children are converting to autism. Yes, *converting*. Most do not have autism at birth.

6. In the case of the autistic child, food is medicine and medicine is food. In every case of autism I've encountered, the child has gut issues.

7. A healthy lifestyle is essential for every child with autism spectrum disorder. Changing will not be *quick-fix*, and will require taking food from the child that he probably loves.

8. It is critical to focus attention on what your child eats and drinks. Fast food, boxed and canned food, dairy, soy, wheat, refined or chemically produced sugars must all be eliminated.

9. It will be necessary to plan your child's meals in advance. This is the only way to control what goes into his mouth.

10. It takes time to make changes. Everything cannot and should not be done at once. It may take as long as six months before all the changes are affected. But if you take one step at a time it will happen. You may see positive results in as few as thirty days.

11. These lifestyle changes will cost money. Organic food is essential. You will have to plan and cook your child's meals yourself for the most positive results.

12. You must do functional lab testing to determine your child's needs, and find answers to why your child is ill.

13. If we band together and wake up to what we are doing to ourselves and future generations through the food we eat we can implement positive changes. Together, we can kick the pervasive Quick-Fix Syndrome. We must accept that there is no silver-bullet solution for the autism crisis.

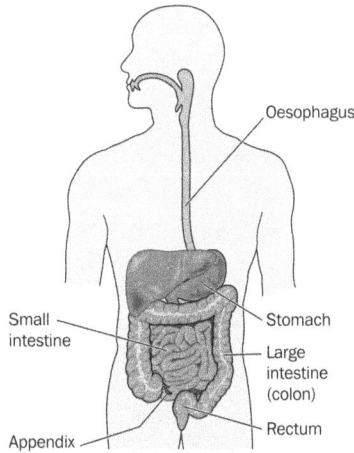

Chapter 2: Autistic Kids Have Sick Guts

The first place we must focus attention is your child's digestive tract—specifically, her small and large intestines. I have found Leaky Gut Syndrome (LGS) in all children labeled "autistic" or "on the spectrum."

This particular phenomenon is confirmed repeatedly through stool samples and functional lab testing. In my years of working with autistic children I have yet to encounter a child that did not have LGS. It causes both child and parent to suffer. If the gut isn't happy, the brain isn't happy.

After confirmation of LGS, which causes your child pain and debilitates her, proper food and nutritional supplements become essential.

Leaky gut syndrome is an itch that cannot be scratched. It is a constant irritation deep inside the body, an extreme discomfort every waking hour of the day. Children with LGS are not comfortable in their own skin. Autistic children have a more difficult time dealing with the uncomfortable sensations. They are in a constant state of agitation and cannot be still.

What is Leaky Gut Syndrome?

Leaky gut syndrome is a condition in which the lining of the small intestine becomes damaged, and allows the passage of harmful substances into the bloodstream normally blocked by a healthy intestinal lining, hence, *leaky* gut syndrome. Spaces form between the cells of the gut wall that shouldn't be there. Bacteria, toxins, undigested food, and waste leak through. The intestinal lining breaks down and degrades. If LGS is severe, the gut will leak feces back into the blood stream casing more severe medical issues.

What Causes Leaky Gut Syndrome?

Poor diet, intestinal bacterial imbalance, parasites, yeast, and prescription drugs can each be the cause. The effective treatment of this disorder is dependent upon the identification of which factors are responsible. Unchecked, the body becomes increasingly toxic and serious illnesses results. In a child with LGS, the lining of the stomach and intestines may allow protein particles to enter the bloodstream, causing immune reactions and chronic inflammation.

Hydrochloric acid (HCL) in the stomach is an essential part of digestion. When the stomach doesn't produce enough HCL, a breakdown of the intestinal lining may occur. There are key minerals and vitamins that assist in hydrochloric acid production. Functional lab testing is able to identify this serious deficiency

> LGS is a complex syndrome that can be caused by many factors. Functional lab testing narrows the possibilities and gives us a place to start.

that causes key minerals to fail to be extracted from food. Low-HCL causes proteins to be improperly digested, creating amino acid shortages that impact brain health and diminish brain function.

There are other contributing factors, too. When a child is under chronic stress, the body is in a constant "fight or flight" mode. This impairs the blood flow to the digestive system, and the stomach and intestines cannot repair themselves. Plus, a diet consisting predominately of processed foods contributes to serious digestive difficulties compounding LGS. Chronic antibiotic use erodes the digestive tract and can set it up for this disorder.

Symptoms of Leaky Gut Syndrome

LGS is often difficult to diagnose in the autistic child who is unable to communicate what she is feeling. Diagnosis of LGS is complicated by the wide variety of symptoms that could be caused by other diseases. However, there are some specific signs to watch out for:

- Diarrhea and constipation
- Constant complaints of stomach discomfort
- Aggressive behavior, hostility, and irritability
- Abdominal pain and swelling
- Brain fog and learning disabilities
- Sick all the time
- Allergies and sensitivities to environment and chemicals

Functional lab testing is the most effective method for diagnosing Leaky Gut Syndrome.

The Healthy Digestive Tract

The intestinal lining has three primary functions:

- It allows for the absorption and transport of nutrients into the blood.
- It is a protective barrier, preventing yeasts, toxins, viruses, bacteria, and undigested food particles from passing into the bloodstream.
- It is an important part of our immune system that fights off viruses and infectious bacteria before they invade our body.

A healthy and functioning intestinal lining has small spaces between the cells. These spaces open and close. They are gatekeepers that allow healthy, necessary nutrients to enter the blood, and prevents unhealthy compounds from passing through.

Waste products and other dangerous substances are kept inside and pushed into the large intestine where water is taken out, stool is formed, and then eliminated.

The leaky intestinal lining allows toxic substances into the blood setting up an immune response—the body thinks it's being invaded by an unknown enemy. This creates sub-clinical, body-wide inflammation which taxes the adrenal glands. Symptoms include irritation, allergic sensitivity to the environment, and a brain that cannot be calm.

Eliminate leaky gut and:
- Allergies disappear.
- Pain ceases.
- Inflammation in joints disappear.
- And many other distresses and dysfunctions stop.

In conjunction with other functional lab tests, analysis of a stool sample provides a clear picture of what's going on in the gut.

Effects of Leaky Gut Syndrome

Once the intestinal lining becomes too permeable:

1. The body can no longer absorb nutrients properly which leads to malnutrition and mineral deficiencies regardless of the nutritional content of the food consumed.

2. Large protein particles, yeasts, dangerous bacteria, and toxins enter the bloodstream. This in turn causes the body to attack them as foreign invaders and sets off a series of *autoimmune*

responses—the immune system becomes confused and attacks healthy cells.

3. In the gut, the immune system loses its ability to protect the body from viruses and bacteria. In a chain reaction, the pathways in the gut which are designed to remove toxins from the body become passive and fail to detoxify the many chemicals we are exposed to on a daily basis. The liver becomes overloaded and is not able to neutralize chemicals and eliminate them safely from the body.

Dealing with Leaky Gut Syndrome

Treating LGS is challenging. Parents must understand that even though this illness is not commonly diagnosed by conventional medical doctors, there is very little a conventionally trained medical doctor (M.D., D.O., etc.) can do anyway, other than prescribe a cocktail of drugs to quell symptoms.

It is more effective to find a professional—most often a naturopath, a Doctor of Naturopathy (ND)—trained to do a full workup on your child employing functional lab testing, who will work in collaboration with your MD. This team approach better serves your child. More likely than not, the Naturopath will also initiate a *specific elimination diet*—described later—to identify foods to which your child is intolerant.

> The bulk of what you feed your child should be healthy, whole foods.

The initial elimination diet determines the foods your child must avoid. Wheat, gluten, dairy, soy, corn, citrus, shellfish, peanuts, and certain other nuts are the most common inflammation-causing foods and should be eliminated from the start to see rapid results.

Healthy, whole foods should comprise the bulk of what you feed your child. All processed food, including *all fast food*, must be eliminated from the diet until LGS symptoms are under control.

- Organic meats, wild-caught fish, organic fruits and vegetables, and gluten-free pastas and grains will give your child's gut the chance to heal.
- Refined carbohydrates and processed sugars must be avoided as they exacerbate negative symptoms, especially if there is yeast overgrowth or a parasitic infection, which is common.
- Appropriate nutritional supplementation can go a long way toward reversing LGS. Only the highest quality supplements will get the job done, and not all supplements are created equal; more about this later.
- Your child's diet will most likely be supplemented with digestive enzymes. Digestive enzymes help break down food, especially protein, essential to brain and body health.

Your child is best served when your pediatrician works in conjunction with the Naturopath, thus utilizing the specialized training in each discipline.

Please note that the advice of your clinicians can only get you started on the right track. The rest is up to you. The most important work that you will do for your child happens outside the offices of your healthcare professionals.

Probiotics

Your child's diet will be supplemented with specific forms of probiotics. Probiotics are the friendly bacteria that help to balance intestinal flora and aid in digestion and absorption of nutrients. The experts agree that a complete regimen of high quality probiotics is necessary to repopulate the intestinal tract and allow the intestinal lining to repair itself. Probiotics promote proper immune secretions which in turn supports the gut. They control overgrowth of yeasts, parasites, and harmful bacteria. They break down acidic bile that can destroy a healthy intestinal lining.

Functional Lab Testing is Mandatory

It is important to understand that only through functional lab testing (FLT) will you be certain of your child's nutritional status. FLT provides specific information not available with other testing methods:

- You will know what foods your child should not eat.

- The supplements and the type of probiotics your child needs will be specified.

- Your healthcare practitioner can design the treatment program that will address your child's *specific* issues.

Cautionary Note: There are methods by which an LGS assessment is made and should be monitored under the direction of a knowledgeable healthcare professional. The content of this chapter is for informational purposes only and should be understood in the context of this book to get a complete and accurate picture of the author's position on LGS and autism.

Chapter Two Summary

1. With autistic kids, the first place to focus attention must be the gut.

2. Leaky gut syndrome is a condition in which the lining of the small intestine becomes damaged, allowing the passage of damaging substances into the bloodstream.

3. There is a mixture of causative factors in the development of LGS. Poor diet, intestinal bacterial imbalance, parasites, yeast, and prescription drugs may be to blame.

4. LGS is often difficult to diagnose in the autistic child who is unable to effectively communicate what she is feeling. However, there are specific symptoms to watch for. Among them are diarrhea

or constipation, constant complaints of stomach discomfort, aggressive behavior, hostility, irritability, abdominal pain and swelling, brain fog and learning disabilities, being sick all the time, and allergies.

5. When the digestive tract is healthy, the lining of the intestines is selectively permeable. It allows nutrients to pass, but prevents yeasts, toxins, large particles of food, and bacteria from entering the bloodstream where they can cause debilitating health issues.

6. In LGS the normal spaces in the intestinal lining become destroyed by inflammation, enlarge, and permit harmful particles to leak from the intestines into the bloodstream.

7. Often, once the gut is addressed, allergies disappear.

8. Treating LGS is challenging. Parents must understand that this condition is not commonly diagnosed by conventional medical doctors, nor does conventional medicine have the tools to effectively reverse it.

9. Healthy, whole, natural foods should be the bulk of what you feed your child. Eliminate all processed food from your child's diet until LGS symptoms are well under control.

10. Appropriate use of *high quality* supplements can go a long way toward reversing LGS.

11. Probiotics are the friendly bacteria that help to balance intestinal digestion and aid in absorption of nutrients. The experts agree that a complete regimen of high quality probiotics is necessary to repopulate the intestinal tract and allow it to repair itself.

12. Your child's diet will be supplemented with digestive enzymes that help break down food and allow the absorption of nutrients from that food.

13. It is important to understand that only through functional lab testing can you be certain of your child's health and nutritional status.

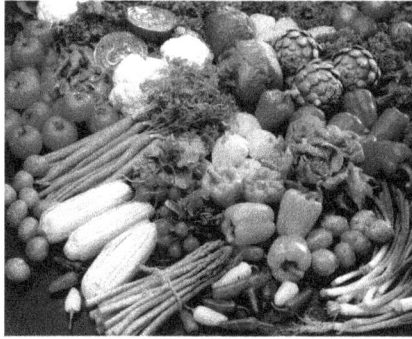

Chapter 3: Food is Your Medicine & Medicine Your Food

What most people think of as *food*, simply is not.

Nowhere has the Quick-Fix Syndrome been more insidious and deadly than the harm we perpetrate on ourselves through what we consume. The old adage, "you are what you eat" is still true, as well as, "garbage in, garbage out." Whether we accept it or not, what we eat is a major contributor to our quality of health. Our choice of food will be a detriment or benefit to future generations.

How we have chosen to eat over the last fifty years is not entirely our fault. We have been duped by the organized food industry into thinking that what they offer us is real food. There are hundreds of millions of dollars spent every year to hide what really goes on behind the scenes in food production. They are spending millions of dollars lobbying Congress to avoid having to list ingredients and the country of origin on your food products. Why, if there's nothing to hide?

> There is no situation in which food awareness is more important than when we're helping an autistic child.

I could go into great detail about how food is produced and makes its way into supermarkets. If I did, you'd never want to put it in your mouth again, and most definitely not in the mouths of your children. But that's not the purpose of this presentation.

However, if you want to understand the industry and politics of food in America, I highly recommend the documentaries, *Food, Inc.,*

Food Matters, and *The Future of Food.* These thoughtfully produced films provide an in-depth view into food production and the billions of dollars generated at the expense of public health and safety.

It's not just about your autistic child; the health of your entire family depends to a very large degree on the quality and purity of the food you eat. Your health is your legacy to future generations.

As a Naturopath, I am committed to educating people about the importance of being mindful, not mindless, regarding what they put in their bodies and calling food.

No place is food awareness more important than when it comes to our autistic children. These kids are gut sick, and food must be their medicine. There is no way to get around this, if you want your child to achieve the maximum in health and wellness.

Back to Food Basics

What is food? Just because it can be eaten, is it food? No. Thanks to *Wikipedia* for providing this comprehensive definition:

*Food is any substance consumed to provide **nutritional support for the body**. It is usually of plant or animal origin, and **contains essential nutrients**, such as carbohydrates, fats, proteins, vitamins, or minerals. The substance is ingested by an organism and assimilated by the organism's cells in an effort to produce energy, maintain life, and/or stimulate growth.* [**Emphasis** added by the author.]

Is it any surprise that food is necessary to maintain life? It's just common sense that food must contain nutrients for life. But much of what's available on our market shelves doesn't fit that definition. It satisfies hunger, and tastes good, but it's devoid of the *essential nutrients* for a *healthy* life.

Food is fresh organic fruits and vegetables. Food is protein from organically raised livestock that has not been saturated with antibiotics, hormones, or themselves fed with genetically modified organisms (GMO) and other non-food substances.

How did America get so far away from the concept of what real food is? How did we come to accept the phony, devitalized, chemical-laden, substances all but devoid of nutrition that are offered to us today? How did we come to believe that this magnificently created machine, the body, could maintain good health and thrive by eating scandalously denatured food? If you follow the almighty dollar in industrialized and technology-based food production, you'll unearth—pun intended—eye-opening clues that provide answers to these questions.

Rich Nation, Poor Health

America is recognized as one of the richest nations in the world, yet we hold the dishonorable distinction of being among the most obese and sick. Each year we rack up a $147 billion dollar medical burden from obesity related diseases and that cost is growing. The number of children and adolescents with Type 2 diabetes has skyrocketed within the last twenty years. For the first time in history, our children may have shorter life spans than us, their parents.

Autism is in that mix with a much publicized dramatic increase in its numbers over the last two decades. It is anticipated to continue growing at an annual rate of ten to seventeen percent, and it has become more common than cancer in our children. Does this not strike fear in your heart? Do you not wonder how the future will look when these autistic kids become autistic adults? And… who will take care of them when their parents are gone?

A Dramatic Change in Our Diets

Beginning in the 1950's our diet changed dramatically from natural farming processes developed over thousands of years to scientific farming processes. There have been more changes in food production in the last fifty years than for the last ten-thousand. Running parallel with this transformation are our fast-paced, stressed lifestyles that have promoted the explosion of quick-fix solutions to mealtime, aka fast foods. This in turn has led to massive food processing changes which have caused unforeseen disease patterns. It's killing us slowly and insidiously, but surely.

Since our need for quick-fix solutions in food preparation and delivery has been responsible for the explosion of the food-industrial-complex, we share some of the blame. We enjoy modern kitchen spaces, yet the microwave oven is the most used appliance.

It has been scientifically demonstrated that microwave cooking destroys many of the most essential nutrients in food. Cooking in a conventional or convection oven is the best way to cook and preserve nutritional content. But it takes more time.

I'm not unsympathetic to parents who have to work and still care for family. I'm in that category. It's a major responsibility and there are only so many hours in the day. So, we fall prey to the Quick-Fix Syndrome.

As a Naturopath, I know that if we don't find the time to provide our families with nutritious prepared food, we are heading down a dark and dangerous path.

Processed Food is Fake Food

Fast food—whether from the drive-thru or boxed meals from the supermarket—has had the nutrition processed out of it. Remember the definition of food? Any food that undergoes changes through processing and is therefore no longer nutritious, is not food. It's fake—a food imposter.

While we may very well be fooled by slick advertisements and eye-catching packaging, our bodies are not. Our bodies know we've been taking in garbage, and the growing trends in disease can be traced to what people have been eating.

> Industrial processing destroys the nutritious properties of food. It may look and taste good, but it provides none of the compounds required for the health of your child's body or brain.

Processed food is manufactured using industrial methods and threatens our health. As of this writing, there is legislation proposed to ban trans-fats—partially hydrogenated oils—which are an unnatural, entirely manufactured substances that have been in our food supply since the introduction of Crisco® in 1911. In recent decades it has become ubiquitous as a preservative and cheap flavor enhancer saving food manufacturers millions of dollars annually—even after it was conclusively demonstrated to cause coronary artery disease in adults and youngsters.

The word *processed* has been bandied about routinely in our society. It refers to procedures that kill the nutritional structure of real food that is vital for our health, but also includes the introduction of non-nutritive, manufactured substances that undermine health.

If you continue to eat non-nutritional food, it will erode your well-being, cause infirmity, and shorten your life.

I keep saying, "It's not food!" However, continually referring to fake food as "food" at all, is a highly effective programming method that has been strategically applied in food marketing and packaging campaigns. It's a way of keeping us duped into believing that we are actually eating something that is life sustaining. I refer to it as "frood" since I consider it erroneous to give denatured food the honorable title "food." Hence, I've coined the term "Frood:" Processed Food = Fraudulent Food = *Frood*.

Frood has been denatured and devitalized, heated, reheated, degraded, adulterated, fragmented, chemically altered, and despoiled until it bears no resemblance whatsoever to a product of nature.

It has been shot full of preservatives so that it can sustain a long shelf life. It has been saturated with coloring to replace its natural color lost in industrial processing. Its packaging makes it look tasty, and most people equate tasty with nutrition; this isn't so. Often there are claims that it is *natural*. This false claim is legal, the product of legislation that gives the food processors the right to lie.

Frood includes everything you get from a fast food restaurant, without exception, including the salads.

Frood is any nonorganic packaged or canned food. By the time it gets in that box or can, or is handed to you through a drive-through window, the nutritive life has been processed right out of it.

Additionally, canning, freezing, and dehydration techniques used in processing destroy most of the food's flavor. Not to worry though, here's where the *flavor industry* comes in. Produced by the same chemical firms that produce industrial pesticides, thousands of chemical flavor formulas have been developed that add back into denatured food the taste you expect.

It's all a fraud that can fool you at the counter, but cannot fool your body or that of your child. I am convinced that among the many diseases and dysfunctions incited by froods is autism.

Get the Full Support of Your Family

Everyone in the family, young and old, can benefit from the same program that we'll design to restore health to your autistic child. And everyone needs to understand that this is a decision that has been made in the best interest of your child. It should be made clear that they have no option but to conform to your requirements. The quality of your child's life depends on it. Once people understand this, they will want to be helpful and do all they can.

> A single *treat* provided by a well-intentioned grandparent could set your child's progress back by weeks.

And here's the challenge. Your family must support you, not your child. An action by a loving grandparent, such as offering your autistic child a little bitty piece of candy, or a tiny piece of birthday cake with a bit of ice cream could slam the brakes on healing, setting progress back by weeks.

No matter how well-intentioned they may be, to ignore your child's program is to extend the time your child spends under the heel of autism.

Chapter Three Summary

1. What we think of as food, is not. Nowhere has the Quick-Fix Syndrome been more insidious and deadly than the harm we perpetrate on ourselves through the so-called *food* we eat. The old adage still holds true: "You are what you eat."

2. There are millions of dollars spent every year to insure that consumers are oblivious to how food is produced. Manufacturers aggressively keep us in the dark about what they are putting into their bodies—what we are eating.

3. If you want to gain insight into the politics of food, view the documentaries, *Food, Inc., Food Matters* and *The Future of Food*. They provide insight into the mechanization of the food industrial complex, which increases corporate profits at the expense of your health.

4. No place is food awareness more important than when it comes to what we feed our autistic children. Autistic kids are gut-sick. Food is

their medicine. There is no way to get around this if you want your child to achieve maximum health and wellness.

5. What is food? What is actually the definition of food? Maybe, somehow along our life paths, we have forgotten, or even worse, been brainwashed into thinking that just because it's called food, and advertised as such, it is food. Not true. *Food is any substance consumed to provide nutritional support for the body. It is usually of plant or animal origin, and contains essential nutrients, such as carbohydrates, fats, proteins, vitamins, or minerals. The substance is ingested by an organism and assimilated by the organism's cells in an effort to produce energy, maintain life, and/or stimulate growth.*

6. America is recognized as one of the richest nations in the world yet we hold the distinction of being among the most obese and sick. For the first time in history, our children are likely to have shorter life spans than their parents!

7. Autism has had a dramatic increase over the last two decades. It is anticipated to continue growing exponentially. Among children, it has become more common than cancer.

8. Beginning in the 1950's, our diets dramatically changed from natural farming processes to scientific farming processes. Running parallel with this transformation are our lifestyles that have promoted the explosion of quick-fix fast food. This in turn has led to massive food processing changes which have led to an outbreak of diseases that are killing us.

9. Fast food is not really food! It is fake food that has had the nutrition processed out of it, and is so highly processed that it is threatens our health! The word "processed" has been bandied about so routinely in our society that many of us haven't really thought about what it means. The important thing to understand is that whenever you hear the word processed in relation to food, it refers to procedures that kill the nutritional structure of the food.

10. Fake food has undergone processing that denatures and devitalizes: heating, reheating, degrading, adulterating, fragmenting, impairing, and chemical altering. It is despoiled until it bears no resemblance to the original product of nature. I refer to it as "frood." Processed Food = Fraudulent Food = Frood.

11. Frood is all fast food served to you from a fast food restaurant, including the salads.

12. Everyone in the family, young and old, can benefit if they were on board and complied with the treatment program that is designed for your autistic child.

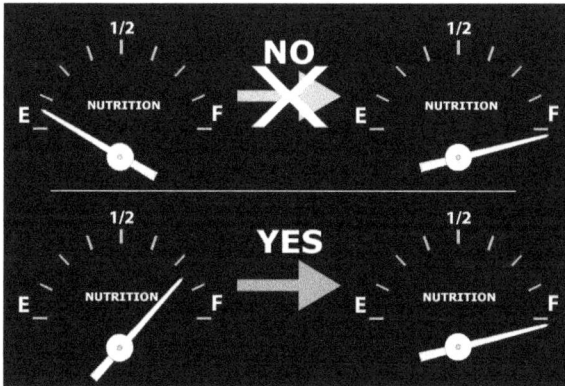

Chapter 4: Supplements

Supplements may be pills, tablets, or liquid preparations. They provide one or more of the vitamins, minerals, enzymes, cofactors, amino acids, and complex nutritional compounds that are essential for a healthy body and mind.

Their purpose, as the title suggests, is to supplement a healthy diet, not to provide these elements as an excuse for an unhealthy diet.

Supplements are a concession to our 21st century lifestyle. What we eat may miss some of the compounds necessary to assure health. Supplements *top-you-off*, ensuring that your body has all of the building blocks and metabolic tools it needs to ward off disease, eliminate inflammation, provide optimum neurological function, and fundamentally slow the aging process.

A Necessary Addition to the Autistic Diet

It is difficult—some would argue that it's impossible—to get the nutritional support our bodies need, even if one works toward a well-balanced, whole food diet without some supplementation. This is a major reason they have become an important part of maintaining health.

Because of their digestive issues, autistic children are particularly prone to nutritional deficiencies. It is essential that they take supplements.

Autistic Children Are Nutritionally Deficient

Autism is linked to autoimmune illnesses and disorders of the gut which lead to abnormal enzyme function, and thus inadequate digestion and nutrient absorption.

> *Key point:* It is not sufficient to provide nutritious food to a child if that child's digestive system cannot absorb that nutrition into the blood stream to be delivered to the cells of the brain and body. Nutritional absorption disorders are almost universal in autistic children.

Autistic kids tend to have very particular tastes in foods. Most prefer to eat the same foods day after day. They refuse to try anything new. These factors set them up to develop food sensitivities and nutritional deficiencies from the start. Even if they do eat healthy, well-balanced meals, they are still at a disadvantage due to their digestive challenges.

Vitamin deficiencies aggravate widespread medical and neurological problems. Wherever your child is nutritionally deficient, the gap must be filled with nutritional supplementation.

> Industrial agricultural practices have stripped our soil of nutrients dramatically reducing the nutritional content of our crops.

The first step is to identify the deficiency. Second, determine why it is happening. This is most accurately achieved with *functional lab testing*, a series of tests that are not commonly employed by medical doctors. More about FLT in Chapter 5.

Research studies by the *Defeat Autism Now! Project* (DAN!), as well as by Tim Buie, M.D. of the Harvard Pediatric Gastroenterology Department, shows that the majority of autistic children have multiple nutritional deficiencies. Supplementation can bring about dramatic changes for many of these children.

The bodily functions of autistic children are different than those outside the autistic spectrum. All the children I have encountered have leaky guts. Since food is largely undigested as it moves through their systems, they are in constant nutrient deficit. It is imperative that these nutrients be replaced with digestible supplements. But what are some of the reasons that we, and not only our autistic children, are so nutritionally deficient and in need of supplementation to stay healthy?

Our Food-Crops Are Grown in Dead Soil

Crops produced in the United States—and *for* the United States—are grown in nutrient depleted-soil. Thus, our food crops lack the life sustaining nutrients and minerals our bodies need to stay healthy. So, how are we getting the nutrients we need? The answer is, we're not.

Industrial agricultural practices have stripped our soil of life-sustaining nutrients and these essential nutrients cannot be manufactured by our bodies. This has drastically reduced the nutritional content of our crops.

As an example, Vitamin A has decreased over forty percent in six items that have been tracked by experts: apples, bananas, broccoli, onions, potatoes, and tomatoes. Since 1951 both onions and potatoes have a complete loss of Vitamin A. To repeat, *industrially grown onions and potatoes produced for the mass market are devoid of Vitamin A.*

There are very few small farms. Industrially produced crops are not rotated, as nature requires, for protection against nutrient-depleted soil, and the soil is not re-mineralized.

Further, the *scientific advances* of the last fifty years have had a devastating impact on the production of food and have set us back nutritionally. Modern farming techniques, introduced during the Nixon administration have resulted in soil erosion, soil compaction, salt intrusion, water logging, destruction of beneficial bio-diversity, and loss of natural enemies of pests that protect crops naturally.

Regarding Genetically Engineered & Modified Food

The interruption of natural growth patterns of crops and the soils that support them is only part of the 21st century, profit-hungry food industry. Genetically engineered (GE) and genetically modified organisms (GMOs)—the health impact of which has already been shown to be harmful to humans—have been foisted upon us without our knowledge.

The 2002 documentary *Fed Up!* states that GE/GMO crops made up major proportions of the 1999 harvest:

- 60% of Canada's canola crop
- 90% of Argentina's soybean crop
- 50% of the American soybean crop
- and 33 % of the American corn crop

…and those percentages are much higher in 2013.

The main GMO crops are soy, corn, canola, and sugar beets. Derivatives of these are found in more than seventy percent of the foods in supermarkets. The primary reason for genetic engineering is so crops will more effectively absorb and retain deadly doses of poisonous pesticides! Industrialized agriculture uses hundreds of millions of pounds of pesticides, and guess where these high toxic residues end up? Inside you!

Fast food, and most non-organic processed foods contain genetically modified ingredients. Every year Big Farm increases the number of GMO foods it sells to unsuspecting consumers.

What about that Fast Food?

Busy families eat frequently at fast food restaurants, putting children's health at risk with large amounts of fats, sodium, MSG, non-nutritive additives, sweeteners, preservatives, food dyes, fillers, and sugar.

Fast food is deficient in dietary fiber and essential micro-nutrients such as vitamins and minerals. To make matters worse, fast foods are guzzled down with sugar-rich drinks.

Reminder: Fast food is hazardous not only to your autistic child, but to you too!

High calorie foods rich in fats, refined sugar, and high fructose corn syrup, reconfigure body chemistry to make you crave these hazardous substances. *Frood is addictive.* Why else would an intelligent, educated person, like yourself, continue eating things you know are unhealthy?

The more you eat, the more you want, and the more you want, the more you eat. How is this different from cocaine or heroin?

It's even worse for autistic children, who become hooked on frood at a young age. Who hasn't picked up a container of fries from the drive-thru just to tide their child over to dinnertime?

The result is that your autistic child—who is more susceptible due to his malady—develops a taste for fatty, salty, artificially flavored foods. It's the same for the mid-day sweets. It is difficult for them to ever develop a taste for health-promoting fruits and vegetables.

Autistic children tend to eat a limited number of foods. If their diet is dominated by fast foods, then they will be nutrient deficient. Nutritional supplementation is absolutely necessary. By first providing your child's body with what it needs, it will be easier—not easy, but easier—to wean your child off a fast food addiction.

What are Autistic Children's Greatest Nutrient Deficiencies?

The following are some important vitamins and nutrients that autistic children often need supplemented:

- Vitamin A: Activates the immune system, supports immune memory, protects against viruses, and is critical for vision, sensory perception, attention-span, and language processing.

- Vitamin B1: Plays an important role in carbohydrate metabolism and biosynthesis of nucleic acids and neurotransmitters. It is also an antioxidant.

- Vitamin B2: Necessary for the building of healthy DNA.

- Vitamin B3: Can have positive effects on cerebral blood flow.

- Vitamin B6: Some autistic children with excito-toxic* damage to brain cells may have a vitamin B6 deficiency.

- Vitamin B12: Deficiencies can cause problems with mental functioning including confusion, slow thinking, forgetfulness, and psychotic episodes.

- Vitamin C: Numerous physical problems develop with a deficiency, including weakness, pain, swelling, rash, fatigue, bruising, and gum disease.

- Vitamin D: Helps transport calcium to cells, along with other benefits.

- Vitamin E: An important antioxidant that scavenges free radicals.
- Folic Acid: Deficiency has been associated with numerous neurological problems.
- Vitamin K: Helps regulate blood coagulation.
- Zinc: Important for brain development and supports the immune system.
- Magnesium: Deficiency can decrease blood flow to the brain and cause symptoms such as sensitivity to sound.
- Calcium: Helps build teeth and bones, plus, it is essential in numerous other biochemical processes throughout the body.
- Selenium: Important for immune protection and critical for pancreatic function.
- Molybdenum: Supplementing can help decrease urinary wasting of important proteins.
- Omega Fatty Acids: Linked to facets of neurological health.
- Essential Amino Acids: All autistic children are lacking in several of these important nutrients that also support brain wellness.

*Excito-toxins, the most common of which is aspartame—the artificial sweetener—cause a disruption of brain function, erratic synaptic communication, confusion, and hyperactivity in people who are not on the autistic spectrum. What damage is caused by feeding your autistic child this unnatural substance?

Supplements Must Be Food the Body Recognizes

Implementing the *elimination diet* is essential. However, purchasing supplements from store shelves using a shotgun approach will result in flushing your money down the toilet—literally.

An important criterion for supplements is that they be recognized by the body as food, so they can be absorbed and not just eliminated in pee or poop. And you don't want to add more toxicity to an already taxed glandular and immune system, a possibility with cheap, industrial, faux-supplements.

Supplements are food and for them to be potent and effective, the body must recognize them as such. This is one reason that your child must take supplements more than once a day. Just as you need to eat several times a day, you also need to take food supplements on the same schedule.

Think of supplements as extensions of each meal. They fortify and correct the imbalances that are revealed through functional lab testing.

Supplements Are Different than Prescription Drugs

A diagnosis is required for a physician to choose a drug appropriate to a disease or dysfunction. The diagnosis is made in combination with conventional lab tests and the symptoms that accompany each disease. This works fine for certain diagnosis: an antibiotic is prescribed for an infection, and medications may be provided for other clearly defined diseases.

But many drugs are designed to eliminate symptoms giving the *illusion* of healing. The danger in chronic drug use is that the body is constructed to be nourished by food, something that comes from the same source as people did, and not a synthetic compound made in a chemical lab—a substance very far from nature.

More serious disease can develop from chronic prescription drug use. Using drugs to suppress symptoms is not getting to the *root cause* of the problem, and prescription drugs simply cannot put an imbalanced system back in balance.

Note: an antibiotic will eliminate the root cause of an infectious disease by killing the bacteria or other invading organisms causing that disease. But they do so only by killing them *faster* than they kill the cells of your body and the beneficial bacteria on which you rely for proper digestion and nutritional balance. As a rapid response to invading bacteria, they are a reasonable treatment. Once antibiotics do their job, you must take supplements and other health promoting steps to recover from their negative effects on your body.

I am not anti-drug. In addition to the case of infectious disease, when one is in a crisis situation, drugs may be necessary to stabilize an out-of-control condition. But that is as far as I believe it should go. Nutritional steps should always be taken in conjunction with supplements that enable you to wean off the drug as soon as possible. Why? Because prescription drugs are chemically manufactured; they are unnatural to the body. While they can serve a useful purpose for crisis intervention, they do not come from nature and should be thought of as useful for short term use only.

Prescription drugs are not natural. There are no Prozac or Nexium® trees. They are developed in laboratories and designed to halt the *red flag alerts* sent by the body in the form of symptoms. Drugs come with a long list of side-effects because, in most cases, they do not treat the disease, they just plug up the symptom—like turning off the fire alarm, but doing little to put out the fire.

Supplements, on the other hand, are food that contain the vital nutrients human bodies require to thrive efficiently and healthfully. Supplements, along with meal-based nutrition, heal the body; symptoms naturally disappear.

Functional labs reveal imbalances that can only be fixed by specific supplements at the right dosages. These lab tests are often repeated within a few months to track progress and to adjust programs accordingly.

Not All Supplements are Created Equal!

Pretty packaging and high price tags do not ensure a quality product. In my practice, I use supplements from a firm I have worked with for more than twenty years. The company has its own FDA approved lab and a drug license. Every batch of raw material received by the lab is tested before it is used. If the raw material doesn't meet their criteria, it is rejected.

This laboratory tests its supplements throughout their manufacture. The finished product is then tested once again for potency. This ensures the efficacy of all ingredients up to the expiration date. What

> While everyone loves a bargain, nutritional supplements that affect your child's health are not the place to scrimp.

appears on the label is actually in the product.

This just isn't so for many supplements and vitamin tablets, including the most popular advertised brands found on store shelves.

While everyone loves a bargain, supplements are not the place where price or marketing should be used as guidelines. The difference in quality between brands is often considerable, and your child's health is in the balance.

The following are five questions you should have answered before buying *any* supplement:

1. Does the company actually make the supplement? Many companies do not manufacture their own products. They merely place their labels on the package and market them. They perform no quality control.

2. Are the ingredients listed on the label actually in the product? You would be shocked at how often they are not. Part of the problem is the way in which supplement companies do business. They use a document called a Certificate of Assay. This document states that the batch actually contains the material. However, most companies don't test batches of material; they rely on this document. There is little impartial or governmental oversight into the practices of these companies. None of the players are required to keep records of the handling of the materials and no one is accountable. *Caveat emptor.*

3. How is the tablet or capsule made? Something as simple as how a tablet is produced can affect bio-availability. Many manufacturers include inert ingredients that interfere with the absorption of the nutrients by the body.

4. How long will the supplement keep its potency on the shelf? This is another *label claims* issue. Vitamins break down over time. Will the label be accurate after six months? A year? Is there a clear expiration date on the vitamins? A good company will put more of each ingredient into the capsule or tablet so that the label claims will be true well past the expiration date.

5. Are the products tested for quality and contamination? The best way to protect yourself is to find a company you trust. One that makes its own products, and tests the quality and purity of its products. You should know where the raw materials come from. Most of the botanicals purchased in America are from the Far East. There are manufacturing practices in third world countries that don't meet the standards Westerners demand.

The Consumer's Dilemma

As a consumer, much of the information you need to answer these questions is difficult to find.

This makes it important to work with a health professional schooled and experienced in the use of supplements. Select someone who does functional lab testing, and can design a specialized program for your child. That person will be able to guide and coach you through the process of selecting supplements and use them to the greatest benefit of your child.

Functional lab testing is the *only* way you can know for certain what supplements your child needs. As harmless as a B6 vitamin might be touted, if given in the wrong dosage or not in conjunction with B-complex vitamins that are able to be used in an autistic child's system, it can cause other issues. If your child has liver, gallbladder, or pancreas issues, as most autistic children do, giving fat soluble vitamins that are bought off a store shelf can create unwanted and dangerous problems. This is just one example of how even simple vitamins can cause issues.

Chapter Four Summary

1. It is difficult to get the nutritional support our bodies need, even from a well-balanced, whole foods diet.

2. Autism is linked to autoimmune illnesses and disorders of the gut which lead to abnormal enzyme function, and thus inadequate digestion and nutrient absorption. This sets autistic children up to be nutritionally deficient from the start.

3. Vitamin deficiencies can cause or aggravate medical and neurological problems. It makes sense that your child's nutritional deficiency requires supplements.

4. Every child I have encountered has a leaky gut. Since food remains incompletely digested, essential nutrients leach out of their

bodies. It is imperative that these nutrients be replaced through supplementation.

5. Crops available in American produce bins are grown in nutrient depleted-soil. This causes food crops to lack nutrients and minerals. This has a devastating effect on the nutritional value of our crops, making it harder to get everything your body needs even at the fruit and vegetable bins of your supermarket. Cost-cutting advances have reducing the nutritional content of our food. Spraying crops with pesticides is not just bad for *our* health, it kills the essential bugs and worms that work with plants to make them nutritious.

6. Agricultural scientists have produced genetically engineered plants or what is more popularly referred to as genetically modified organisms (GMOs). This process has made the food industrialized complex more profitable at the expense of your health.

7. In the 2002 documentary *Fed Up!*, it was revealed that a major proportion of our food crops are genetically modified, even though it has been demonstrated that GMOs are dangerous to humans.

8. Recent scientific studies have shown that high calorie food rich in fats, refined sugar and high fructose corn syrup, artificial flavorings, and salt, reconfigures body metabolism in such a way that you crave foods that are hazardous. Fast food has become addictive.

9. Nutritional supplements are essential, however purchasing supplements from store shelves often results in you flushing your hard earned money down the toilet.

10. Quality nutritional supplements are recognized by the body as food; they are absorbed and utilized. Low quality, indigestible supplements create more toxicity in your child's already taxed system.

11. Supplements are designed to change the expression of genes to promote health. Prescription drugs oftentimes stimulate genes to express themselves in disease forming ways, hence, side-effects. Supplements are designed to promote wellness and longevity. They provide the nutrition that we are not receiving from today's food.

12. *A cautionary note:* This is an informed process that requires training and experience. Work with a qualified professional to determine the supplements your child needs. Select a health

professional that does functional/biomedical lab testing, and who can design a specialized program for your child, and is willing to guide and coach you through the process.

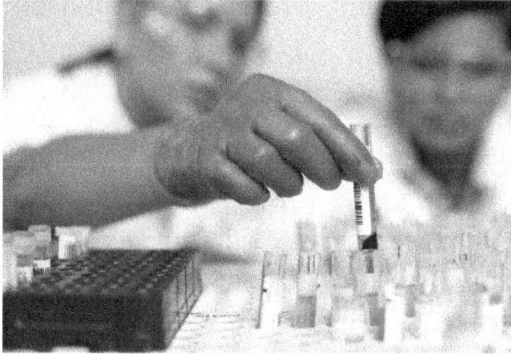

Chapter 5: Functional Lab Testing Provides Answers

In conventional medicine, the average health care clinician isn't able to spend as much time as she would like with patients. This poses a serious problem for those needing to find out what is wrong with them. A forty-five minute office visit that includes only five minutes with the doctor and forty minutes in the waiting room can be harmful to your health. Quick-fixes in terms of healthcare, invariably lead to long term chronic illness.

I have found it impossible to spend less than one hour with each of my clients. My goal is to spend whatever time is necessary to uncover the root cause of their discomfort, often continuing after office hours and after my client has left.

What is Functional Lab Testing?

Functional lab tests are biochemical tests. They detect vitamin, mineral, and other nutrient deficiencies that go undetected with most conventional medical testing. The intent of functional testing is to determine how to help the body heal itself with the application of proper nutritional support.

FLT allows a practitioner to determine which systems in your child's body are not functioning at ideal levels. Once testing has established areas of dysfunction, the professional creates a customized supplement and nutrition-based road map to better health for your child.

Functional Lab Testing vs. Static (Conventional) Testing

What makes a lab test *functional?* When I look at test results, I'm not looking to diagnose a disease or illness. Instead I'm looking for ways to achieve balance and wellness. I'm looking at these tests in combination with your child's history and symptoms to see what systems of his body aren't performing at optimum levels. From there, I'm able to suggest specific adjustments and lifestyle changes that need to be made. The lab results give me the information to determine what supplements need to be added in your child's diet, and what dosages are required to move your child's body systems towards full function. Once all of your child's systems begin to move closer to healthy levels of functioning, symptoms begin to disappear.

My job with functional lab testing is not to find a diagnosis for your child—a medical doctor is licensed to do that. As a Naturopath, I identify the systems in your child's body that aren't functioning at their best, and educate you about changes you can make to help restore optimal health. I do not get caught up in trying to get rid of symptoms directly. My focus is to find the root cause of your child's discomfort and eliminate it. In that way, symptoms disappear.

Most conventional medical lab tests are static. They are designed to show a *snapshot* of the body at a moment in time. Nutrient levels fluctuate drastically from day to day—perhaps even during a day—depending on diet, stress, and other factors. Conventional lab testing does not provide an accurate measure of a person's nutritional status. Static testing may provide results that direct you to a quick-fix pill, but that will never get to the root cause of your child's autistic behavior.

If You're Not Testing, You're Guessing

*Each child is different. The only way you can determine your child's **current status** is to establish baseline information and work from there.*

Time and time again parents tell me that they have taken their child to a number of healthcare practitioners and they still have no positive results. They are frustrated, and their child has suffered all manner of testing and blood work. Parents are anguished because they have seen little progress. Those that have done their homework—as you are, by reading this book—feel that if they could only find out what is causing their child's problem, they could get a handle on making them well.

They've jumped from one program to another without a definite plan of action and no positive outcomes. They're tired of being told, "I don't know." There's a constant outpouring of money, and still, the outcome for their child is unknown.

> At this time, there's no alternative to Functional Lab Testing.

This is where functional lab testing proves to be of tremendous benefit to parent and child. The tests reveal what is going on in your child's body, then a specified program can be developed to target your child's challenges.

No matter what you do, if you're not testing you're guessing! Functional lab work takes the guesswork out of how treatment should proceed, provides your child's *biochemical status*, and gives you the answers to the "whys."

Perform Functional Lab Testing Early

What I've outlined should help you understand why the first approach *must* be functional lab testing, to which there is no alternative at this time.

Next, adopt and adhere to the supplement and nutritional protocol suggested by your health practitioner. Save time and money by implementing your practitioner's plan for your child as soon as possible. Supplements play a significant role in turning a child's issues around. In conjunction with nutritional food, this has proved to be most effective in helping autistic children.

Your child's condition will change over time, and testing needs to be performed periodically to gauge the effectiveness of specific supplements. The test indicates the supplements needed to affect the internal environment of your child's body to produce desired outcomes.

When a rocket is launched to the moon, it needs mid-course corrections to reach its destination. The same holds true for programs I design. Periodic testing gives us the information to tweak the treatment program to move in the right direction.

As I've said before, there is no quick-fix solution; your child's health requires dedication and patience.

Most Health Insurance Will Not Pay for Functional Lab Tests

Tests can be costly because they are not covered or only partially covered by most health insurance companies. However, while these tests appear to be expensive in the beginning, you could end up paying much more in the long run by a conventional hit and miss approach—and still not help your child.

Don't get caught up enrolling your child in an endless stream of therapies, still running the risk of never getting to the root cause of the symptoms. Even worse is staying the course—doing nothing different in the hope that what you've been doing will somehow suddenly become effective. This just doesn't happen. The problem your child is experiencing will not and cannot resolve on its own. Hit and miss approaches often involve buying costly supplements that don't work; these purchases end up being dumped in the trash can.

> Most parents will do what they have to do once they understand the possibility of positive results for their child.

I am aware that there are many people who cannot afford the cost of functional lab testing. I don't mean to sound insensitive; I know they can put a serious dent in your household budget. But I've found that *most parents will do what they have to do* for the overall well-being of their children to ensure they grow into productive, independent adults. Most parents are willing to make the sacrifices necessary *once they understand the possibility of positive results.*

Functional Lab Tests Are an Investment in Your Child's Future

This investment in your child's health and well-being will have lifetime benefits.

No one wants to pay for dental braces, but we do because in the long run it's in our child's best interest. Braces are expensive and it often takes years for teeth to be corrected. Of course, it is just as important for your child to be able to function and enjoy his life; is that not the right of every human being? We find a way, whatever it takes, to help our children regardless of the sacrifices.

When you proceed with testing, you begin to change a sick child into a well child. It is unlikely that an FLT will come back *normal* when there are overt signs of imbalances; your money will not be wasted.

I understand that couples need to talk this over. One or other of a couple often needs more convincing; don't be afraid to ask for assistance from your healthcare professional. If it is necessary for a reluctant parent to have a consultation with the practitioner to gain insight and understanding, this should be done. That parent's objections should be addressed and dealt with to the parent's satisfaction. It's not unreasonable to want to understand why the testing needs to be done, and the outcome that is expected as a result.

Comprehensive Functional Lab Testing for Autism

I use specific tests I believe get to the root causes of the autistic child's issues. Over time, functional nutritional inadequacies can result in a variety of chronic health conditions. Functional labs help determine the basis for complaints and symptoms. The following are the key testing areas on which I initially focus. Some of this gets technical, but I'd rather provide you with too much information than not enough.

There are many functional lab tests. I employ only those specific to the conditions I have come to understand are associated with autism and related challenges.

Test #1 – Stool Sample

Since all of the autistic kids with whom I've worked have some form of gut or digestive issues, a stool sample is imperative. I request a test that provides an accurate picture of the state of the microbiota in your child's gut. I'm looking to identify the imbalances of the dominant bacterial groups in the gastrointestinal tract. This test reveals how well food and fat are being digested and absorbed. It indicates the level of inflammation, and the presence of parasites, yeast, and fungal overgrowth. It identifies the specific organisms that are causing your child problems.

This test identifies drug resistant genes, a huge development in the protocol to health. If an antibiotic is required for a stubborn organism, we'll know precisely the medication to which it's sensitive.

The test has a *biomarker* for gluten sensitivity. There's also a biomarker that identifies the body's primary immune defense deficiencies. Leaky gut and an overall lowered resistance to any infection are identified. Does your child have frequent bouts of strep throat that ultimately cannot be treated with medications? Your child can be continuously re-infecting herself from the gut. This test answers your question, "Why does my child get sick so frequently?"

With just this one test, information essential to helping your child is gleaned. A very precise program can be designed to get the gut healed—a giant leap forward.

Test #2 – Food Sensitivity

It is only through this testing that we can focus on those foods which cause inflammation in your child's gut. That is, those things he's eating that is causing his Leaky Gut Syndrome.

When identified, these are the foods to be eliminated. Without this test, a family would pretty much find themselves having to cut out a long list of suspect foods: the harsh and notorious *elimination diet*. Short of this test there is no way to know what your child is sensitive to.

Test #3 – Combination Profile
- Organic Acids: reveals the nutritional and metabolic basis of symptoms, including anxiety, mood changes, and immune responses.
- Amino Acids: determines essential amino acid imbalances that effect both physical and mental function.
- Nutrient and Toxic Elements: identifies a toxic burden, which can render considerable damage to the brain and nervous system as well as the sufficiency of nutrient elements.
- Fatty Acids: helps strike the right balance of fatty acids that can impact health and development.
- Antioxidant Vitamins: measures a total body status of antioxidant nutrients and nutritional deficiencies.

- Coenzyme Q10: measures total body status of this antioxidant nutrient and energy pathway cofactor.
- Lipid Peroxides: measures total serum lipid peroxidation, an indication of whole body free radical activity.
- Homocysteine: identifies total homocysteine in plasma. Elevated levels are an independent risk factor for premature cardiovascular disease and atherothrombotic cerebrovascular disease.

I recommend all three tests for autistic kids. Rapid progress can be made when this is done. If we start out in this manner I have all the information I need right from the start. It allows me to move the process forward smoothly and almost every element of guesswork is taken out of the equation.

The investment for all three tests outlined above is about $5,000—as of this writing. *(Yes, I actually told you the cost of something without you having to go to a website and register and give me all your personal information. Mom and Dad, I'm serious about your child's health.)*

I understand that finances may not permit the ideal case: performing all three tests at the outset. There are other functional lab options that can be implemented. If money is very tight, at least Test #1, the stool sample, should be performed so we can see what's going on in your child's gut.

> What is the cumulative cost in a single year of lost time and wages due to the special care required by your child?

Chapter Five Summary

1. In conventional medicine, health care clinicians are not able to spend as much time as they would like to with patients. This poses a serious problem for those needing to find out what is wrong with their children.

2. Functional lab tests can detect vitamin, mineral, and other nutrient deficiencies that commonly go undetected with conventional medical testing. The philosophy behind this testing is based on helping the body help itself with the application of proper nutritional and supplemental support.

3. What makes a lab test functional? When I look at lab test results I'm not looking to diagnose a disease or illness. Instead I'm looking at these tests in combination with your child's history and symptoms to see what systems of her body aren't functioning at optimum levels. The lab results tell me what supplements need to be added in your child's diet to move his body systems towards ideal function.

4. Most conventional medical lab tests are static. They are designed to show a *snapshot;* a single moment in time. Nutrient levels fluctuate drastically from day to day depending on diet, stress, and other factors, therefore conventional lab testing does not provide an accurate measure of a person's nutritional status.

5. Each child is different and the only way to determine your child's current status is to establish baseline information and work from there.

6. If you're not testing you're guessing! Functional labs take the guesswork out of how treatment should proceed. It provides the information needed to assess your child's biochemical status. It answers the "Whys?" as it relates to your child's issues.

7. What I've outlined should help you to understand why Functional Lab Testing must be the first approach with your autistic child.

8. FLT is costly; tests are not covered—or only partially covered—by most health insurance companies.

9. You can get caught up involving your child in an endless stream of therapies, and never get to the root cause of the symptoms. Even worse is to choose to do nothing in the hope that what you've been doing will somehow become effective. This just does not happen.

10. Functional lab testing is an investment in your child's health and well-being that has lifetime benefits. When you order functional lab testing, you take a significant step toward your child becoming well. At the very least, it will give you answers that no one else has been able to provide.

11. I use specific functional lab tests that I believe are beneficial in helping me get to the root causes of your autistic child's issues. Over time, nutritional inadequacies can result in a variety of chronic health conditions. Functional labs can help determine the basis for complaints and symptoms.

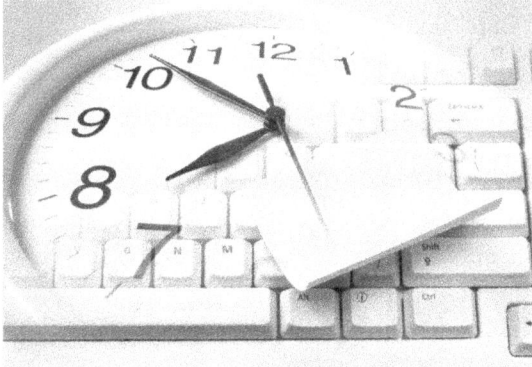

Chapter 6: The Custom Designed Protocol

We've discussed food, supplements and functional lab testing. Now we have arrived at the part of the journey that makes my heart sing. It is the critical juncture where I do what I enjoy most and what I do best—custom design a supplement protocol for your child. The development of your child's plan to health takes a lot of time and focused energy. For optimal results the program must be meticulously developed on a month-by-month basis.

Any thoughts of quick-fix solutions must be thrown out the window. Patience is required. However, you will be glad you persevered when you see the results reflected in your child, often in the first thirty days.

When You've Decided to Proceed

You are taking positive action to improve the quality of life for your child and family, and I am here to support and help you every step of the way. To see your child, who could not be still for one minute, and who was plagued with seizures, become calm and have a significant, perhaps complete, reduction of these episodes is gratifying. Your family will have the opportunity to relax and enjoy each other without the overriding daily stress experienced in caring for a totally dependent and sick child.

These only scratch the surface of the marvels I've seen in working with autistic children.

The Path to Recovery Has Been Established

I want to provide a clear picture of what to expect. When a family is ready for me to design a protocol, three things have already happened:

1. *The initial office visit.* I have met with the parents or guardian who has completed a detailed questionnaire regarding the child's symptoms. I've spent at least an hour observing and evaluating the child's complaints and issues. I've determined the parents' objectives and explained the detailed plan to health that needs to be implemented.

2. *Functional lab tests have been ordered.* The family has decided which functional labs they choose to have performed. When the sampling kits from the testing lab arrive in the mail, detailed instructions take you step-by-step through the stool, blood, and urine collection process. Once submitted, test results come back in three to four weeks.

3. *The hypo-allergenic/anti-inflammatory diet has started.* You have been instructed to begin this diet immediately. You should not wait until you receive test results.

I keep the big picture in mind; what we want to accomplish is clear. Gut issues are the first I address. As stated earlier, one hundred percent of the autistic kids with whom I've worked have inflamed, poorly functioning digestive tracts. Once their gut begins to heal and your child can better assimilate proteins, fungal and parasite issues are addressed. Then we can focus on their body/brain system as a whole.

The Hypo-Allergenic/Anti-Inflammatory Diet

You begin the **hypo-allergenic/hypo-inflammatory diet** (HA/HI). It must be part of your child's daily routine. The process of introducing whole, natural foods into meals is launched. The following is an outline of the diet:

HA/HI Diet Basics—Foods to Avoid

- All gluten-containing foods including wheat, rye, oats, and barley are eliminated. These are found in breads, box cereals, pasta, and other products of refined flour. The most common allergies and sensitivities autistic children experience are caused by this group of foods. By avoiding these for a few weeks, their system relaxes and clears out. You may not even know that your child has sensitivity to these foods, because symptoms may be subtle and are often delayed for days after eating the offending food.

- No caffeine containing foods (coffee, black teas, chocolate, sodas). No soy milk or any soy product, carbonated drinks, or fruit drinks that are high in refined sugar and high fructose corn syrup. This is important for the benefit of the adult members of the family who also intend to benefit from this cleanse. For them, no alcohol either. Both alcohol and caffeine are hard on your liver. Give your liver a vacation!

- No pork, cold cuts, bacon, hot dogs, canned meat, sausage or shellfish. Nitrate free, organic hotdogs and lunch meats are okay—these are seasoned with sea salt. *Applegate* and *Niman Ranch* are among brands that offer these products. Meats, unless organic, are typically high in nasty ingredients such as xenoestrogens, antibiotics, nitrates, MSG, and other poisons, that are neurotoxins. These are typical of processed foods.

- No corn or tomato sauce, though whole, fresh tomatoes are okay. These are common allergens and can contribute to pain and inflammation.

- No dairy: milk, cheese, yogurt, butter, etc. Dairy products are likely to cause allergies and can increase pain and mucous congestion. Stay away from salad dressings such as ranch and creamy garlic, as they contain dairy. But a small amount of organic butter is okay.

- No foods high in fats and hydrogenated oils, including peanuts, refined oils, margarine and shortening, reducing the burden placed on the system.

- No refined sugar products, candy bars, or other junk foods. Refined sugar slows the process of detoxification weakening the immune system. It is a neurotoxin!

- Of course, avoid all other foods to which you know your child is allergic or sensitive.

Begin the elimination diet while waiting for the test results. This gives you three to four weeks to get your child—and family— accustomed to major food changes before we introduce supplements.

It is important to *clear out your food cupboards.* Get rid of the foods that your child cannot eat. I know this seems harsh but it is necessary. I've had many experiences where a child was doing very well, their gut healing, their behavior much improved, with seizures reduced or absent. Then *zap*, everything seems to fall apart and the parents call me in a panic. Each time, we traced the regression back to something the child got a hold of that they shouldn't have. Nine times out of ten it was an item hidden in the back of a kitchen cabinet that, if it had not been there, the child could not have gotten. Is it worth running the risk of setting your child back weeks, when he or she is doing so well? Throw it out.

> If it's not in the house, it can't be offered. Even a single bit of prohibited candy or junk food given by a well-meaning grandparent can set your child back weeks. Why risk it?

Make It a Family Affair

When the entire family embarks on what we're doing for your autistic child, the whole family benefits. Siblings get healthier, too. This is the reason it's a good idea for the entire household to go on the food elimination program. You can make it a family project in which everyone participates for at least ninety days.

I know many families that have done this and they were pleased and amazed at how much better *everyone* felt. It was worth making the sacrifice so their autistic child wouldn't feel excluded. It also makes it easier on parents who won't have the added burden of preparing separate meals. Often, mom and dad find that they are *getting along* better as well.

Time to Go Food Shopping

Unless you already have your family on a whole, natural food diet, it's time to go food shopping. Wherever possible you should buy organic food. Here are some helpful suggestions:

16 Ways to Transition to Organic Foods *on a Budget*

1. Gradually transition to organic. Start out buying organic versions of some of your favorite foods. This is essential for the children.

2. Do research. Go online and check out websites such as *Organic Kitchen*, *Organic Consumers Association* and *Eat Well Guide*. Here you will find many links to information about organic foods. They are also good resources for you to find organic foods in your local area.

3. Look for sales and house brands of organic foods. Organic awareness is growing and merchandisers are competing for "organic dollars." Be alert for discount fliers offered by your favorite market and grab them at every opportunity. When your favorite organic food is marked down, stock up on it. Don't overlook house brands. Any food with the words "USDA organic" on its label must go through the same certification process regardless of its brand name. Buying organic house brands can save you money.

4. Look for coupons. Organic foods sold under the brands *Cascadian Farm*, *Amy's,* and *Muir Glen* often carry coupons on the inside of their packages. Look online for coupons offered directly from the manufacturer.

5. Get to know your local farmers' market. You can find great sources of fresh, local produce at farmers' markets. Buying at these markets is actually one of the best kept secrets to buying affordable, organic food. A just-picked tomato from a local farm tastes better than a tomato that's traveled thousands of miles before reaching a supermarket shelf.

6. Feel free to ask question of farmers at the market. Farmers like talking about their produce and will often provide tips on what they think tastes best. Don't pass up misshapen fruits or vegetables—ugly veggies—just because it doesn't look like a magazine advertisement.

They will be absolutely delicious, nutritious, and very gentle on your wallet.

7. Don't rule out nonorganic when it comes to local farmers. Get to know the farmers. Look them square in the eye and ask, "Do you spray your food?" Let them know you have an autistic child or a child on the spectrum. Let them know the importance that this question be answered truthfully. You will become a loyal customer to them. A lot of the meats they offer come from grass-fed animals that are humanely slaughtered. It's not rude to ask questions, questions, questions.

8. Join a co-op. This can save you money and provide local access to organic produce. A food cooperative is a member-owned business that provides groceries and other products to its members at a discount. Many of the products found in these grocery stores are organic and much of the produce comes from local family farms. To join the co-op, you sign up by paying yearly dues, often just a few *Latte equivalents*. To locate a co-op near you, check out websites such as *LocalHarvest* and *Cooperative Grocer*. If you don't find a co-op in your area you can start your own. You can get a how-to brochure from Cooperative Grocers' Information Network.

8. Buy a share in a community-supported agriculture (CSA) program. You help a local farm's operating expenses and in return, you receive seasonal fresh vegetables and fruits weekly from the harvest. This is a good way to rotate your fruits and vegetables.

You don't get to pick and choose; you get whatever is available in the current harvest, but it is well established that the healthiest way to eat fruit and vegetables is to eat what is in season, as nature intended. A share in a CSA could cost $300 to $400 upfront for a half-year growing season. Many CSA programs accept weekly or monthly payments, and you may be able to buy a half-share rather than a whole share. Check websites such as *Alternative Farming Systems Information Center*, *Food Routes,* and *LocalHarvest* to find a CSA closest to you.

9. Grow your own organic garden. This is a great way to save cash. Grow organic tomatoes, lemons, limes, bell peppers, lettuce, cucumbers, squash, herbs and other produce that would otherwise be added to your grocery bill. It's a good idea to grow the most

expensive organic produce of those you enjoy. This is also a great way in involve your child as she awakens from her challenge. The entire family will enjoy eating what they've grown.

If you live in a small space you can try container gardening. You can find seeds at companies like *Seeds of Change. The Organic Kitchen* has many useful organic gardening tips.

10. Join a buying club. A buying club is a good way to get the organic food you want at a reduced price, perhaps thirty to forty percent off retail. Buying-club members purchase food and other organic products in bulk and then split the stash. Ask a co-op near you about starting a buying club with your friends and neighbors. Some co-op grocers allow you to order directly from their store. You can contact a local natural food store and ask them where they get their items and contact the distributor directly. Some distributors will deliver directly to individuals or groups.

11. Rethink your food budget. You can free up more dollars for organic food by cutting back on your conventional food budget. Add up all the dollars you spend every month on food, including fast food meals, morning cups of coffee, bagels and trips to vending machines. You'll be surprised how much you can save by eliminating some of these items, especially the junky fast food that's not as cheap as it was many years ago. Gradual changes in your eating habits could free up the money you need to buy the organic foods that you enjoy and are much better for your health. You can find some tasty organic food recipes at *OrganicAuthority.com.*

12. Use a grocery list. Although this may seem obvious, you'd be surprised how many people don't do it. Studies show that people who use grocery lists save considerably on their grocery bill.

13. Buy organic coffee and tea. If you must have that coffee or tea, drink organic brands. Organic crops of coffee beans and tea are grown without harsh chemical fertilizers or toxic pesticides. Make sure that the brand is "shade grown" as this guarantees that age-old, earth-friendly techniques are used.

14. Buy in bulk. Buying in bulk is a great way to stretch your food dollar, whether you shop at a supermarket, natural foods store, or co-op. For beans, grains, lentils and nuts, look for the bulk containers.

It's important that you have a cool, dry place in your kitchen to store your dry goods for a few months.

15. Buy fruits and vegetables in-season. Buying fruits and vegetables in season is best because the prices are lower due to abundant supply. It's also the best time to buy in large quantities. Load up on all your favorite organic fruits and veggies at dirt-cheap prices and consider freezing them. There are lots of resources online that give great tips on freezing and canning if you choose this money-saving practice.

16. Commit to dining out less. In my opinion, going through a drive-through window, even if it's just once a week, is one time too many, and it's not cheap anymore. If you must, choose healthier fast food establishments. You can check online for the listings of the healthiest fast food restaurants. If you scale back eating fast food from four or five times weekly to just once or twice, that's great. You'll have more money in your pocket and you'll also find more room in your budget to buy quality foods that are tasty and nutritious while supporting a healthier family. No matter how convenient you think it is, if you go through that drive-through window you're taking a serious negative hit to your health. Both your budget and your waistline will thank you.

Pesticide Contaminated Foods

It is healthiest to choose locally-grown, organic produce when possible.

The top twelve on the following list are the "Dirty Dozen." Minimize cost by purchasing organic versions of these which are among the most contaminated. You could reduce your overall pesticide exposure by up to eighty percent.

Then, as your budget allows, expand your organic-only purchasing.

Pesticide Contamination of Fruits and Vegetables

Rank	Food Item	Score
These are items highest in pesticide contamination: seek Organic		
1 (highest)	Peaches	100
2	Apples	93
3	Bell Peppers	83
4	Celery	82
5	Nectarines	80
6	Strawberries	80
7	Cherries	73
8	Kale	69
9	Lettuce	67
10	Grapes – Imported	66
11	Carrots	63
12	Pears	63
13	Collard Greens	60
14	Spinach	58
15	Potatoes	56
16	Green Beans	53
17	Summer Squash	53
18	Peppers	51
19	Cucumbers	50
20	Raspberries	46
21	Grapes – Domestic	44
22	Plums	44
23	Oranges	44
24	Cauliflower	39
25	Tangerines	37
26	Mushrooms	36
27	Bananas	34
28	Winter Squash	34
29	Cantaloupe	33
30	Cranberries	33
31	Honeydew Melon	30
*These are items are low in pesticide contamination: Conventional is okay		
32	Grapefruit	29
33	Sweet Potatoes	29
34	Tomatoes	29
35	Broccoli	26
36	Watermelon	26
37	Papaya	20
38	Eggplant	19
39	Cabbage	17
40	Kiwi	13
41	Sweet Peas – Frozen	10
42	Asparagus	10
43	Mango	9
44	Pineapple	7
45	Sweet Corn – Frozen	2
46	Avocado	1
47 (lowest)	Onions	<1

This list was compiled by the Environmental Working Group from approximately 96,000 USDA and FDA studies between 2000 and 2008. There are many fruits and vegetables that are not on this list. These were chosen because they are the most commonly eaten.

The hardest part of the new lifestyle will be implementing the dietary restrictions. Having foresight for unexpected contingencies will make your job a lot easier and this can only be accomplished if you have the right food on hand. While the car can ebecome an extension of the pantry, it is best to plan meals and save even more time and dollars by not having to run out to the grocery for just one thing.

The Elimination Diet is a Detoxification Process

The process of cleaning up your food is a form of detox. If you've ever tried to give up caffeine, you know that the first day you feel terrible. You get a headache, you feel sluggish and you are irritable. This feeling may stay with you for a number of days until your body adjusts to the lack of caffeine; you're in a form of withdrawal, a detoxification process.

If you notice your child's behavior getting worse after starting the elimination diet, it's a good sign. It demonstrates that imbalances do indeed exist. Be prepared for your child to—perhaps—throw temper tantrums. This is not easy for him, but some tough-love is required. Take heart. This will be temporary and there is light at the end of the tunnel.

A lot of the restricted foods are the ones that are craved by autistic children—and all children—who are addicted to them. Foods that are sugary and highly processed feed yeast and parasites. When the supply stops, these organisms die off, and various forms of aberrant behavior can be promoted. The first few days are the worst but if you stick with it the withdrawal symptoms taper off and you will see positive changes. Tuck and roll!

You will see changes in bowel habits. Your child could experience constipation or diarrhea. This is a sure sign that you are addressing imbalances in the gut.

On the flip side, positive signs such as decreased agitation and reduced hyperactivity will occur; your child becomes more focused and calmer. If she has had seizures, there will be less seizure activity. Bowel habits will normalize.

As we continue along the elimination diet path, we are waiting for the functional lab test results.

The Functional Lab Results Have Arrived!

The elimination diet should have been in place for at least three weeks. Now it's time to evaluate test results and determine what supplements your child needs.

Designing and implementing this part of the protocol is a labor-intensive process. I spend a considerable amount of time evaluating labs which are comprised of biomarkers that reveal specific nutritional imbalances. It's a complex puzzle that I assemble.

I design the first thirty-day protocol of a month-by-month program. Because each child is different, only now do I know for sure what supplements your child requires.

If test results show that her gut is severely compromised we may have to focus our efforts with some basic GI-tract support. The supplements required to heal and rebalance an unhappy gut may be more than a child can tolerate. Again, this is the beauty in testing; I look to the test results to decide what comes first and what comes next in a measured and orderly progression. As her gut heals, we can reduce the supplements for this issue and address other deficiencies.

Operating in the Real World

Have you ever had a major street or highway—one you use every day—get closed down for roadwork? Often it can be blocked off for quite a while. It's an inconvenience—okay, it's a royal pain. Life gets tougher. We do what we have to do. We have no choice. Eventually, a newly paved, perhaps widened roadway is opened and your commute is easier and faster than it was before.

> Unlike prescription medications, no harm can come from this approach.

I have witnessed the challenge of getting an autistic child to take supplements three times a day. I understand that it's easier for some than others, but it must be done. We watch to see how your child responds. I'll discuss this in more detail in Chapter 7, but ultimately a child, family, and lifestyle emerges that is better than you could have thought possible.

Tweaking the program—mid-course correction—is an ongoing process. Sometimes we find that we have to proceed slowly. Other times we move full speed ahead. It depends on your child's reaction.

The good news is that no harm can come from this approach. We may have to slow down if your child has stomach issues due to rapid detoxification. We simply stop the supplements for a couple of days and start again more slowly. Once his system gets strong enough, it will better tolerate the supplements at the dosages that are needed.

As his immune system gets healthier and stronger, his body will tell us what comes next. It may reveal that deeper imbalances exist. We're peeling back the layers of an onion to uncover the root causes of bodily discomforts. It may be what we anticipated or something unexpected. Either way, we deal with it.

We test. We implement the food program. We incorporate the supplements into your child's daily routine. Your child enjoys results in the first month. By the end two months... well... you'll see. But you've got to keep things going for at least ninety days, and then, not lapse back into fast food hell or it will all be for naught.

Some Final Thoughts on Alternative Therapies

It's up to the clinician to make the educated and informed decision as to what comes first. For example, I have seen a lot of parents jump right into any number of alternative therapies. This can be a mistake because if the gut and biliary system are not healthy you will not get good results. Your child needs a healthy gut first.

We are building up his immune system, strengthening glands and organs—liver and kidneys—whose role is to detox the body. When you move cautiously and slowly, better results follow.

Chapter 6 Summary

1. The development of your child's plan to health takes a lot of time and focused energy. There is no quick-fix solution; patience is required. When you see positive results reflected in your child with the first thirty days, you will be glad you persevered.

2. Gut issues are the first addressed. Autistic kids have inflamed guts. Once healing starts, other specific issues are addressed. Then we focus on the system as a whole.

3. It is time to begin the hypoallergenic/hypo-inflammatory diet and ensure it's included in your child's daily routine. You introduce whole, natural foods into your child's meals.

4. You start the elimination diet while waiting for test results. This gives you three to four weeks to get your child accustomed to major food changes before we introduce supplements.

5. Clear out those food cupboards! This is important. It's best to get rid of the foods that your child cannot eat, so there is no chance that they'll be found, or a well-meaning grandparent won't slip your child a bit because "Just a tiny bite can't hurt." It can and will!

6. When the whole family is involved in helping your autistic child, the whole family benefits. It's a good idea for the family to go on the food elimination program together as a family project; everyone participates for at least ninety days. I know many families that have done this and they were both pleased and amazed at how much better *everyone* felt.

7. Shopping: wherever possible buy organic. I provide you with sixteen ways to transition into organic foods on a budget.

8. The hardest part of the new lifestyle will be implementing the dietary restrictions. Having foresight for unexpected contingencies will make your job a lot easier and this can only be accomplished if you have the right food on hand.

9. The process of changing food is a form of detox, something a lot of people do not realize.

10. If you notice your child's behavior getting worse after starting the elimination diet, that's a good sign. At the beginning of their road to health, be prepared for your child to throw tantrums. Take heart. This will be a temporary stage and there's light at the end of the tunnel.

11. On the flip side, parents begin to see positive signs such as a reduction in agitation and hyperactivity; your child becomes more

focused and calmer. If he has had seizures they are fewer and less intense. Bowel habits normalize.

12. When lab results are received and evaluated, specific supplements are suggested.

13. Designing and implementing this part of the protocol is a labor-intensive process in which I spend a considerable amount of time evaluating lab tests. Biomarkers reveal specific nutritional imbalances, and I design the first thirty-day protocol of the month-by-month program.

14. The good news is that no harm can come from this approach. We may have to slow it down if rapid detox causes stomach issues such as diarrhea. We simply stop the supplements for a couple of days and start again slower. Once your child's system gets stronger, it can better tolerate the recommended dosages.

15. As his immune system gets healthier and stronger his body tells us what comes next. It may reveal that deeper imbalances exist. We're peeling back the layers of an onion to get to the root causes of discomfort. It may turn out to be something totally unexpected, or we may have been spot-on from the beginning.

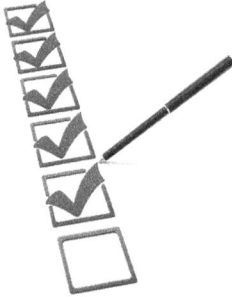

Chapter 7 – Compliance is the Key to Success

By now you understand the fundamental role of food in achieving and maintaining long term health. There should be no doubt in your mind that most autistic-spectrum kids have very sick guts—you likely know this from personal experience.

You grasp why functional lab testing is essential to draw a roadmap to health based on your child's nutritional deficiencies. You also understand the crucial role that supplements play in the healing process. You appreciate how the specifically designed protocol ties all the factors for healing together.

Once a comprehensive plan is in place, your emphasis must shift to the essential key to success—***compliance***. Compliance means that you must follow the specialized program that has been established for your child. Without compliance the organic food on which you spend your money will not be as effective as it should be. To some extent, sick guts will remain inflamed and function poorly. Your investment in functional lab testing will be wasted without compliance. The carefully designed protocol will be for naught and all your efforts—and money—up to this point will go down the drain.

Worst of all, without compliance, your child will never achieve the healthy, quality life that he or she deserves.

But It Doesn't Have to Be All or Nothing

I used to be hard-nosed about compliance. I wanted so much to turn the child's suffering around that I'd be frustrated when there were setbacks due to parents straying from the program. I have since learned that it doesn't have to be all or nothing. The reality is that *life happens* and that you, as already overtaxed parents, are doing the best you can with a very difficult situation.

I'm satisfied with parents taking any baby-steps possible on the long journey to healing their child. I am humbled by the fact that you are willing to spend the money and embark on this challenge to the entire family. It's enough that you've taken the big step of becoming aware and mindful of what you're feeding your child and the affect it has.

I have adopted a more relaxed and compassionate approach, and have adjusted my protocols accordingly. I still recognize that the goal is to get back to simple eating of organic whole food and it's still important that your child eats no fast food, preservatives, dyes or food additives. But there will be times when this is not possible. *The key, when you stray, is to get back with the program as soon as you can.* Don't think that just because a mistake was made and your child deviated from the program that all is lost. On the other hand, don't use one slip up—a single bad meal or snack—as an excuse to blow off an entire day of healthy practices. Just pick up where you left off, do the best you can, and go from there.

Remember, *tuck and roll.*

Your Child Will Not Like the Changed Lifestyle

Your child will likely resist the menu changes you implement. If they don't, you're lucky as this is rare.

Massive dietary changes are necessary. Most everything your child loves will be taken away. It's no wonder that many parents initially balk at adopting such a plan. What they need to embrace is the confidence that their child has a good chance for a much improved quality of life.

What about Those Temper Tantrums?

The question is not whether your child will have a temper tantrum it's "When?" You should expect and be prepared for some meltdowns at the beginning stages of the program. The following tips may prove to be helpful.

What to Do During a Temper Tantrum:

- Remain calm during the entire period of the tantrum. Your facial expressions will be closely observed by your child. Your child continuously takes the cues from your body language. Make sure you wear a calm reassuring face.

- Safety is the most important issue. Make sure your child is not hurting herself by banging her head or body on a hard or rough surface. Make every effort to move the child to a safe place.

- During the temper tantrum your child won't listen, so say only the strictly necessary words. You cannot instruct a child during this crisis situation. However, the child can respond to visual cues.

- Ignore the behavior and walk away if you are at home, and make sure the child is safe to be left on her own. You can position yourself in a location where you can observe the child but where she cannot see you.

- Try to eliminate or minimize the cause of the tantrum. Of course if the tantrum is because you will not give the child candy she wants, you cannot cave in.

- Try to divert the fixation of the child, and direct her attention and interest to something else in which you know she's interested. You need to be positive and calm and show a lot of interest or enthusiasm in what you are suggesting.

- Love helps.

Sometimes an ounce of prevention is worth a pound of cure. The best way to prevent a tantrum is to prepare ahead of time. If you're not prepared, you can easily get caught in the trap of rewarding the undesired behavior. In the middle of the crisis we tend to give in to a child's demands, or promise something we never intend to provide—we lie. If you have an advanced plan of action, you won't be caught by surprise and can move smoothly into *plan B*.

It's not easy to foresee a tantrum, but if you know your child well, you can avoid some of the triggers. Keep your child away from circumstances you know will upset her, especially during the initial stages of the new program. Your child is going to be under stress from having to make lifestyle changes. You don't want to add anything to the equation that you can avoid.

Don't assume that your child understands everything you say or do. It helps to explain how things will change in terms your child might understand. Use real objects, pictures, or written words to help her visualize the new plan. It takes patience, time and effort, but it's worth it if it prevents a temper tantrum.

Don't Skip the Supplements

Although I've relaxed my approach to compliance, what I do insist upon is that the supplements be taken according to the designed protocol. Supplements are your child's new medicine and if taken properly and consistently they will adjust her body chemistry.

It isn't easy to get your child to swallow pills, but it can be done. Supplements are a lot smaller than the size of chunks of food our kids swallow with each meal. How many times have our kids swallowed things like a Lifesaver? If you act casual about it, children are more likely to mimic your attitude.

Here are some tips that I've found to be useful and some I tried with success when my daughter was five years old:

- Speak to your child about what you want her to do, and how she has no difficulty swallowing other food. Explain the necessity for taking the supplements—that it will make help them feel better. Don't worry about whether they understand every word. Just speak in a casual and calm tone, and be relaxed and matter-of-fact about the whole process. If you act like it's no big deal they're more likely to adopt the same attitude. It will take practice but they will eventually get the hang of it.

- If you take supplements, even just a vitamin, take them along with your child.

- You can put one supplement at a time in applesauce (organic) and feed it to them. They can swallow it along with the applesauce.

- Some parents find it helpful to get a mortar and pestle and crush tablets into powder form. Then add it to unsweetened fruit juice, or make a healthy smoothie containing the supplement.

- If you have to put powdered supplements in a tablespoon of raw honey to get your child to swallow it, do it!

- Take your child to your local dollar store and allow her to select a number of little toys. Load up a bag of goodies they really like to play with. Then, when it comes time to take those supplements and they do it, they get to pick a toy from the *goodie bag*. Remember to reward them immediately after they've taken their supplements.

I know you get the picture of how important it is to establish and maintain compliance with your child's supplements. They are right up there in importance with your organic, whole food.

If your medical doctor prescribed a medication that was essential to your child's survival, you'd comply. You would find some way to ensure that the medication was administered at the appropriate times and at the appropriate dosage. Supplements are as instrumental in helping your child. Never think of it as an option to skip supplements. They are your child's "medicine."

When You Can't Avoid Cheating

Realistically, there will be times you're caught short and you cannot avoid cheating. Life happens. If you recognize this in advance and prepare for it you can get your child through it with the least amount of damage.

11 Healthy Ways to "Cheat"

1. I commented earlier that your car can become an extension of your pantry. I was not trying to be flippant. Most often, cheating is necessary when you're caught away from home. Also, your child—and for that matter, you—shouldn't go more than a few hours without a healthy snack. Meals need to be within a four hour time frame.

2. Find the healthiest "fast food" restaurants in your home area so you'll know where they are when you're in a bind.

3. Always have some gluten-free hamburger buns that you keep with you in your car. Choose the best fast food restaurant from which to

get a hamburger, *minus* the condiments, mayo, and special sauce. Throw away their bun and put the patty on your gluten free bun.

4. A good substitute for those fast food French fries are organic potato chips or organic GMO-free popcorn with sea salt. Snack packs are available at most health food stores. Keep a couple stashed in your car.

5. There will be birthday and holiday parties. If you prepare in advance, you can overcome the bulk of the challenges. Make a gluten-free cake or cupcakes and take them with your child to the party. Your child will be just one of many with special dietary requirements or food restrictions. These treats can also be found at healthy foods markets if, like me, you don't bake. Ice cream might be a bigger problem. You can make your own with coconut milk, or buy organic sorbet. If this proves to be a huge problem, allow your child a portion, but try to restrict the amount. Understand that your child's body will pay the price, and you'll have to deal with the aftermath. If you can't prepare, and you know your child will eat regular cake and ice cream, have digestive enzymes specifically designed to handle gluten and lactose on hand. Give them to your child in advance. Ask for assistance in finding these in health food stores.

6. Be prepared for your child to demand cookies and treats. Health food stores have a variety of tasty gluten-free cookies and coconut macaroons. Just make sure you buy organic. Buy a number and try them yourself. Stock up on the ones you believe your child will most likely enjoy.

7. Choose healthy alternatives to candy bars. In the baking section of your health food store you will find Sunspire—a brand name— chocolate covered drops; they're like M&Ms, but they have no food dyes in their shell. This company also makes dark chocolate chips that can be added to the chocolate drops for a nice candy mix. Put the mix in baggies and make them your child's new *candy bar*. Purchase only dairy-free and be sure to read the labels to avoid forbidden ingredients.

8. There are healthy alternatives to cold cut meats. You will find companies that make nitrate free roast chicken, and ham or turkey

bolognas. *Applegate* and *Niman Ranch* are two that are widely available.

9. Although I recommend avoiding canned foods due to potential metal leaching, wild caught salmon is an option to widen the diversity of foods you prepare. *Do not use tuna* as it is high in mercury, a substance anecdotally associated with autism. Still, fish is problematic because of ocean contamination, so serve it only on occasion. Common fish with less contamination include haddock, hake, flounder, pollock, wild Pacific salmon, speckled trout, white fish, wild Atlantic salmon, herring, smelt, sardines, and anchovies. If through taste-testing you find that your child is not sensitive to shellfish, you can include clams, shrimp, scallops, and lobster. Examples of fish to avoid are swordfish, albacore white tuna, shark, king mackerel, and orange roughy. Avoid farmed fish, which, like feedlot-raised cattle and poultry, are typically fed unnatural foods in crowded conditions that make them susceptible to sickness.

10. Make your own popsicles from organic unsweetened fruit juice. You can purchase the molds at any supermarket. My daughter used to love them.

11. Be manic about reading labels. Do not purchase anything that contains high fructose corn syrup, corn syrup solids, partially hydrogenated oils, trans fats, MSG, or artificial flavorings or colors. There are many companies that make stevia-sweetened carbonated drinks if you must give one to your child.

Fine Tuning With the *Diet Check Record*

Your child's *Diet Check Record* is instrumental in tracking your child's responses to the foods he eats. I have a form that I provide to my clients when they begin a program. You record your child's good and bad reactions to their food. It breaks the reactions down into categories: appetite, satiety, cravings, energy levels, mind, emotions, and well-being. It is formatted so that all you have to do is √ your child's responses after each meal or snack.

There are some basic rules to remember:

- Write it down: Keep the form with you, and write down *everything* your child eats and drinks.

- Do it now: Don't depend on your memory at the end of the day. Record what your child is eating as the day goes along, and his reaction to it.

- Be specific: Make sure you include *extras,* such as gravy on meat and anything put on their vegetables. Do not generalize. For example, record a bag of potato chips as a bag of potato chips, not as chips.

- I tell parents that a dinner sized plate is to be used as a pie chart. Each meal will be a combination of animal protein, vegetables, carbohydrates and fats. It is important to remember that fats are not just vegetable oils, butter, etc., they're also found in lean meat.

Example: On your dinner sized plate you put about 30% meat, you calculate 25% fat (knowing there is some fat in most meat), and the rest will be vegetables and carbohydrates (pasta, rice, etc.) 45%. I start with these percentages of food combinations and make adjustments if necessary.

Keeping a good Diet Check Record will enable you to fine-tune your child's food choices until every food he
.eats becomes healing medicine.

It Gets Easier and Better With Time

It is a mistake to think there is a quick-fix solution to turning your child's issues around. If you allow yourself to entertain thoughts like this it will only frustrated you. What I'm recommending is definitely not a quick-fix journey. It can sometimes take months and even up to two years to get *everything* corrected. It depends on how sick your child is. But it does get easier and better with time.

The good news is that with help your child's body will begin the healing process and you will rejoice at the outward expression of a happier child. His system will clean out, and when you have that occasional dietary *faux pas,* his body will do some screaming. You will understand that the protocol is on the right track. You'll wonder, if one transgression can wreak havoc on his body, how he tolerated what you were doing to him every day. You will understand why, once upon a time, your child was so sick.

It's okay to ease into the program. We're not trying to win a race; we're getting your child healthy. Don't feel you have to do everything at once. If you start with your first step by focusing on breakfast everyday and making it the healthiest organic meal, free of additives and preservatives, that's okay. Making breakfast the perfect meal is a major start. Then you can graduate to lunch and dinner until you've included the whole day.

Chapter Seven Summary

1. **Compliance** means following the specialized program that has been established for your child. Without compliance the money spent on organic, whole foods will go to waste. Your child's sick gut will remain inflamed and nonfunctional. The functional lab tests in which you've invested will do your child no good. The carefully designed protocol will be for naught and all your efforts will go down the drain. Worst of all, without compliance, your child will never achieve the healthy quality life she deserves.

2. Compliance doesn't mean all or nothing. Life happens. Just do the best you can in a very difficult situation.

3. A major dietary change is required. Your child is not going to like the lifestyle changes that you implement. Many things your child loves to eat must be removed from her diet.

4. The question is not whether your child will have a temper tantrum, it's "When?" You should be prepared for some meltdowns at the beginning stages of the program.

5. Sometimes prevention is worth a pound of cure. The best way to prevent a tantrum is to prepare ahead of time. You can easily get caught in the trap of rewarding undesired behavior if you're not prepared. Don't be caught off guard; move smoothly into *plan B.*

6. Don't assume that your child understands everything you say or do. It helps to explain what's going to happen. Use real objects,

pictures, and written words to help visualize what he has to do. It takes patience, time and effort, but it's worth it if it saves you a temper tantrum.

7. Sometimes it's necessary to relax compliance, but supplements must be taken according to the designed protocol. Supplements are your child's new medicine and if taken consistently they will improve your child's body chemistry.

8. It's not always easy to get your child to take supplements but it's doable. Pills and tablets are smaller than the chunks of food they swallow. Never think that missing supplements is an option. They should be thought of as medicine, and they are instrumental in helping your child.

9. Use the *Diet Check Record.* It is important to track your child's response to foods with regard to appetite, satiety, cravings, energy levels, mind, emotions, and well-being. Keeping an accurate Diet Check Record will enable us to fine-tune your food choices until every food becomes healing medicine.

13. It's okay to ease into the program. We're not trying to win a race; we're trying to get your child healthy. Don't feel you have to do everything at once. If you start with your first step by focusing on breakfast everyday and making it the healthiest organic meal, free of additives and preservatives, that's okay.

14. Comply with the program for as long as you can. Occasionally, if you need to take a mental break by getting a fast food meal, then so be it. But keep those occasions to a minimum, and keep them in the bank. Don't use them up frivolously. You and your child have a lot to accomplish.

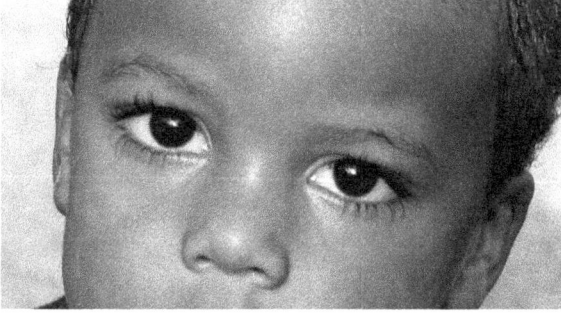

Chapter 8: Tomorrow's Face of Autism

We are in the midst of an autism epidemic—a full blown crisis for our children and our society. There are many that vehemently deny this. However, the CDC estimates that the number of children in America that have autism spectrum disorder has grown to one in one-hundred-ten. If this number of our children developed cancer, there would be a Manhattan Project initiative to find out why.

The ever increasing statistics for autism should be a warning that we are headed down a dangerous path that demands serious evaluation. Our quick-fix solutions, including covering up symptoms with medications rather than making better food choices, have been instrumental in the deterioration of our health as a nation.

If we are to halt the effects of this devastating syndrome, we must pay attention to the nutritional health of our children. We move forward by being aware of the harm we are doing through the non-nutritional, adulterated, processed food we serve.

I view autism as the worst possible outcome of how we have chosen to live. To be as sick as we are, it's apparent that we have little regard for our nutrition. Adults pay the price with late-in-life diseases: unnecessary debilitation we call "just getting old." But our children pay the price soon after their birth, and autism is a wakeup call.

Healthful lifestyle changes are the key. If we don't change the eating habits of our children, as the statistics predict, the autism epidemic will spread.

The Aging Face of Autism

There are even bigger challenges on the horizon within the autism crisis. To date, most of our focus has been on *children* stricken with autism and finding ways to cope with this devastation so they can lead more productive lives. We are now forced to give more thought of how autism will affect future generations. I've often asked, "What will happen to these children when they grow up?" With the ever-increasing numbers of kids on the spectrum, this becomes a scary proposition indeed.

In 1943, seven decades ago, the first article about a condition "unlike anything reported so far" appeared in a medical journal. It was about a boy named Donald T. and was referred to as "Case 1." He was the first given a diagnosis of autism. The crux of the article dealt with what comes next for children like Donald. What will happen to them when they grow up?

Back then, there were only twelve autistic children. The article referred to them as a "wave of children with autism."

If twelve is a wave, the only word for what's happening now is *tsunami.* The statistics are in: within a decade, more than 500,000 of those diagnosed with autism will enter adulthood.

Family challenges will be more pronounced. It's a never ending job for parents whether the child is 5 or 50, but what will society do with these adult children when their parents are gone?

- More than 80% of adults with autism, ages eighteen through thirty, still live at home.
- Unemployment is 81% among adults with autism.
- 78% of families are unfamiliar with agencies that could provide assistance.
- At least *half a million* children with autism will become adults by 2023, and they will need caretaking, housing, food, clothing, and a future.

These are astonishing statistics. The question that haunts every parent of a child with autism is, "What will happen when I die?" inasmuch as *autism does not fundamentally affect a person's longevity.*

Children with autism outlive the parents who have always provided their support. There are estimated to be 88,000 such adults today and their parents all face the anxiety that hundreds of thousands more will confront.

Government won't help. Our system is already hampered by budget cuts. We're not even able to handle the increasing tide of *children* diagnosed with autism; adults will be on their own.

However, we can preempt that tragedy by planning to help our children while we are here to support them.

What We *Can* Do

In the first seven chapters of this book, I've made my case based on my observations and experiences. In a nutshell, we can get ourselves and our children healthy.

I do not have all the answers; no one does. There's no denying that our society is very "sick" and we need to do something about it. Certainly, no harm can come by embracing nutritious eating habits. Consider this *food for thought*:

- We must think in terms of autism prevention, starting with potential parents. Couples planning to have children—both women and men—need to establish a sustainable, healthy lifestyle before conception. If parents-to-be have already adopted a lifestyle of nutrition and health, then mothers will be providing a healthy environment for their unborn children, and once born, kids will learn proper eating habits as they grow.

- Functional lab testing is not just for kids and not just for the sick. Couples planning to become pregnant should invest in testing to determine where they stand nutritionally. They should see what environmental toxins are floating around in their bodies: plastics, toxic minerals and heavy metals, inflammatory hormones, and others. With this information they can embark on a wellness program to balance out their deficiencies and get rid of the toxins in their systems.

- Schedule single-dose vaccines for your children on a schedule that won't stress their developing immune systems. Remember, a child's immune system does not fully develop until the age of seven. You can strengthen the immune system before and after each vaccine.

The unsubstantiated issues surrounding the MMR vaccine controversy is a good reason we should proceed with caution. Know that you have the right to order single dose measles, single dose mumps, and single dose rubella vaccines. There is single dose *everything;* you just have to ask for it and do your research.

This is an important topic to discuss when interviewing a prospective pediatrician. Remember, this approach may very well not be covered by insurance, and you have to be prepared and willing to pay out of pocket.

There is No Quick-Fix, America

The focus of this book has been the growing number of children diagnosed with autism in America, but this epidemic has spread to all industrialized western countries, those that have followed America's fast-food and quick-fix lead.

It took America seventy years to get to today's crisis. It's going to take years for it to be corrected. It may take several generations to fix autism just as it took several generations to create it. But we have to start somewhere. What I've recommended in this book reflects my opinions and what I consider to be viable first steps.

America, please take a good look at these children. Really look. Realize that it's time for us to *wake up.*

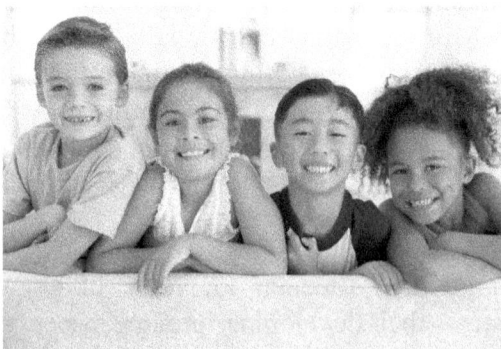

Links to References and Resources

Dr. Brooks' web site & blog: http://AlternativeMedicineAtlanta.net

Contact Dr. Alison Brooks: NatOpt1@gmail.com

The following are websites that I have found helpful. The brief description that follows each reference is from their websites.

Organic Kitchen
http://www.OrganicKitchen.com

Organic Kitchen™ is an organic foods product, research and marketing company, and a registered brand and trademark in the United States of America. We explore the Internet and provide links to websites we think will interest you. In the future, we may make our products available for purchase.

Organic Consumers Association
http://www.OrganicConsumers.org

The Organic Consumers Association (OCA) is an online and grassroots non-profit, 501(c)(3), public interest organization campaigning for health, justice, and sustainability. The OCA deals with crucial issues of food safety, industrial agriculture, genetic engineering, children's health, corporate accountability, Fair Trade, environmental sustainability and other key topics. We are the only organization in the US focused on promoting the views and interests of the nation's estimated 76 million organic and socially responsible consumers.

Eat Well Guide
http://www.EatWellGuide.org

Eat Well Guide® is a free online directory for anyone in search of fresh, locally grown and sustainably produced food in the United States and Canada. The Guide's thousands of listings include family farms, restaurants, farmers' markets, grocery stores, Community Supported Agriculture (CSA) programs, U-pick orchards and more.

Local Harvest

http://www.LocalHarvest.org

The best organic food is what's grown closest to you. Use our website to find farmers' markets, family farms, and other sources of sustainably grown food in your area, where you can buy produce, grass-fed meats, and many other goodies. Want to support this great web site? Shop in our catalog for things you can't find locally!

Cooperative Grocer

http://www.CooperativeGrocer.coop

Cooperative Grocer is a bi-monthly trade magazine for food cooperatives in North America. At *Cooperative Grocer*, our mission is to improve professionalism and mutual education among food cooperative directors, managers and staff, and key allies of food cooperatives. We aim to be a voice of practitioners, the people and organizations that are doing the work of governing and operating excellent food co-ops. The emphasis of *Cooperative Grocer* is on how to learn from others about improving co-op store operations and governance.

About the Author

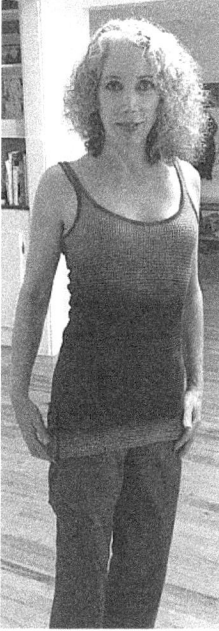

Alison Brooks is a Traditional Naturopathic Doctor living in Metro-Atlanta where she has had an established private practice for almost two decades.

In working with autistic children, her specialty is designing individualized nutrition and supplement protocols based on the results of Functional Lab Testing.

Her successes are borne out by the many laudatory comments she's received from those she's helped whose comments are included in this work.

But Dr. Brooks does more; she walks her talk and maintains a lifestyle in which she keeps fit and eats well. Now into her fifties, she is a model for her patients and all she meets.

Hundredth Shire
Publishing
LLC
http://HundredthShire.com

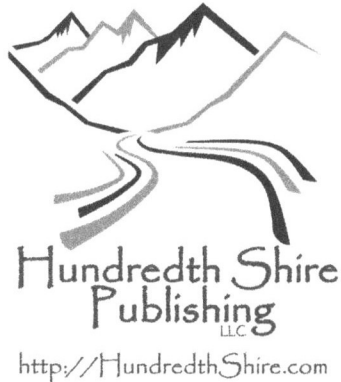

Hundredth Shire Publishing is a boutique press that encourages novel non-fiction and fiction with realism. We seek authors who challenge institutional authority with wisdom and fact, and who weave tales that impact lives.

Founded in 2013, our initial goals are to develop a library of non-fiction in the health, nutrition, and wellness genre. The fiction we promote will be supported by a central pillar of enlightenment that encourages personal and spiritual renewal.

No work is too general or specific to be considered, nor are quality works in other areas.

www.ingramcontent.com/pod-product-compliance
Lightning Source LLC
Chambersburg PA
CBHW030027290326
41934CB00005B/512